Frederic P. Miller, Ag
John N

Kawasaki disease

Frederic P. Miller, Agnes F. Vandome, John McBrewster (Ed.)

Kawasaki disease

Skin, Mucous membrane, Lymph node, Blood vessel, Tomisaku Kawasaki, Heart, Paracetamol, Ibuprofen, Myocardial infarction

Alphascript Publishing

Imprint

Permission is granted to copy, distribute and/or modify this document under the terms of the GNU Free Documentation License, Version 1.2 or any later version published by the Free Software Foundation; with no Invariant Sections, with the Front-Cover Texts, and with the Back-Cover Texts. A copy of the license is included in the section entitled "GNU Free Documentation License".

All parts of this book are extracted from Wikipedia, the free encyclopedia (www.wikipedia.org).

You can get detailed informations about the authors of this collection of articles at the end of this book. The editors (Ed.) of this book are no authors. They have not modified or extended the original texts.

Pictures published in this book can be under different licences than the GNU Free Documentation License. You can get detailed informations about the authors and licences of pictures at the end of this book.

The content of this book was generated collaboratively by volunteers. Please be advised that nothing found here has necessarily been reviewed by people with the expertise required to provide you with complete, accurate or reliable information. Some information in this book maybe misleading or wrong. The Publisher does not guarantee the validity of the information found here. If you need specific advice (f.e. in fields of medical, legal, financial, or risk management questions) please contact a professional who is licensed or knowledgeable in that area.

Any brand names and product names mentioned in this book are subject to trademark, brand or patent protection and are trademarks or registered trademarks of their respective holders. The use of brand names, product names, common names, trade names, product descriptions etc. even without a particular marking in this works is in no way to be construed to mean that such names may be regarded as unrestricted in respect of trademark and brand protection legislation and could thus be used by anyone.

Cover image: www.PureStockX.com
Concerning the licence of the cover image please contact PureStockX.

Publisher:
Alphascript Publishing is a trademark of
VDM Publishing House Ltd.,17 Rue Meldrum, Beau Bassin,1713-01 Mauritius
Email: info@vdm-publishing-house.com
Website: www.vdm-publishing-house.com

Published in 2010

Printed in: U.S.A., U.K., Germany. This book was not produced in Mauritius.

ISBN: 978-613-0-72768-0

Contents

Articles

Kawasaki disease	1
Skin	6
Mucous membrane	11
Lymph node	13
Blood vessel	20
Tomisaku Kawasaki	22
Heart	23
Paracetamol	31
Ibuprofen	44
Myocardial infarction	52

References

Article Sources and Contributors	80
Image Sources, Licenses and Contributors	83

Article Licenses

License	85

Kawasaki disease

	Kawasaki disease
	Classification and external resources
	Kawasaki disease
ICD-10	M 30.3 [1]
ICD-9	446.1 [2]
OMIM	611775 [3]
DiseasesDB	7121 [4]
MedlinePlus	000989 [5]
eMedicine	ped/1236 [6]
MeSH	D009080 [7]

Kawasaki disease (also known as **lymph node syndrome**, **Mucocutaneous lymph node syndrome**[8], and **Kawasaki syndrome**) is a disease, largely of infants, which affects many organs, including the skin, mucous membranes, lymph nodes, and blood vessel walls, but the most serious effect is on the heart where it can cause severe aneurysmal dilations. Without treatment, mortality may approach 1%, usually within 6 weeks of onset. With treatment, the mortality rate is less than 0.01% in the U.S.[9] There is often a pre-existing viral infection that may play some role in pathogenesis. The conjunctival and oral mucosa, along with the epidermis (skin), become erythmatous (red and inflamed). Edema is often seen in the hands and feet and the cervical lymph nodes are often enlarged. Also, some degree of fever is often noted.

It was first described in 1967 by Dr. Tomisaku Kawasaki in Japan.[10]

Signs and symptoms

Symptoms

Kawasaki disease often begins with a high and persistent fever that is not very responsive to normal treatment with paracetamol (acetaminophen) or ibuprofen. The fever may persist steadily for up to two weeks and is normally accompanied by irritability. Affected children develop red eyes, red mucous membranes in the mouth, red cracked lips, a "strawberry tongue",[11] iritis, keratic precipitates (detectable by an ophthalmologist but usually too small to be seen by the unaided eye), and swollen lymph nodes. Skin rashes occur early in the disease, and peeling of the skin in the genital area, hands, and feet (especially around the nails and on the palms and soles) may occur in later phases. Some of these symptoms may come and go during the course of the illness. If left untreated, the symptoms will eventually relent, but coronary artery aneurysms will not improve, resulting in a significant risk of death or disability due to myocardial infarction (heart attack). If treated in a timely fashion, this risk can be mostly avoided and the course of illness cut short.

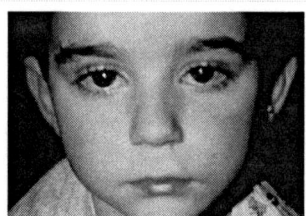

Red eyes and dry, red lips.

- High-grade fever (greater than 39 °C or 102 °F; often as high as 40 °C or 104 °F) that normally lasts for more than 5 days if left untreated.
- Red eyes (conjunctivitis) without pus or drainage, also known as "conjunctival injection"
- Bright red, chapped, or cracked lips
- Red mucous membranes in the mouth
- Strawberry tongue, white coating on the tongue or prominent red bumps (papillae) on the back of the tongue
- Red palms of the hands and the soles of the feet
- Rash which may take many forms, but not vesicular (blister-like), on the trunk
- Swollen lymph nodes (frequently only one lymph node is swollen), particularly in the neck area
- Joint pain (arthralgia) and swelling, frequently symmetrical
- Irritability
- Tachycardia (rapid heart beat)
- Peeling (desquamation) palms and soles (later in the illness); peeling may begin around the nails
- Beau's lines (transverse grooves on nails)
- may find breathing difficult.

Complications

The cardiac complications are the most important aspect of the disease. Kawasaki disease can cause vasculitic changes (inflammation of blood vessels) in the coronary arteries and subsequent coronary artery aneurysms. These aneurysms can lead to myocardial infarction (heart attack) even in young children. Overall, about 10–18% of children with Kawasaki disease develop coronary artery aneurysms with much higher prevalence among patients who are not treated early in the course of illness. Kawasaki disease and rheumatic fever are the most common causes of acquired heart disease among children in the United States.[12] [13]

Causes

Like all autoimmune diseases, the cause of Kawasaki disease is presumably the interaction of genetic and environmental factors, possibly including an infection. The specific cause is unknown,[14] [15] [16] but current theories center primarily on immunological causes for the disease. Evidence increasingly points to an infectious etiology,[17] but debate continues on whether the cause is a conventional antigenic substance or a superantigen.[18] Children's Hospital Boston reports that "[s]ome studies have found associations between the occurrence of Kawasaki disease and recent exposure to carpet cleaning or residence near a body of stagnant water; however, cause and effect have not been established."[13]

An association has been identified with a SNP in the ITPKC gene, which codes an enzyme that negatively regulates T-cell activation.[19] An additional factor that suggests genetic susceptibility is the fact that regardless of where they are living, Japanese children are more likely than other children to contract the disease.[13] The HLA-B51 serotype has been found to be associated with endemic instances of the disease.[20]

Diagnosis

Kawasaki disease can only be diagnosed clinically (ie. by medical signs and symptoms). There exists no specific laboratory test for this condition. It is difficult to establish the diagnosis, especially early in the course of the illness, and frequently children are not diagnosed until they have seen several health care providers. Many other serious illnesses can cause similar symptoms, and must be considered in the differential diagnosis, including scarlet fever, toxic shock syndrome, juvenile idiopathic arthritis, and childhood mercury poisoning (acrodynia).

Classically, five days of fever[21] plus four of five diagnostic criteria must be met in order to establish the diagnosis. The criteria are: (1) erythema of the lips or oral cavity or cracking of the lips; (2) rash on the trunk; (3) swelling or erythema of the hands or feet; (4) red eyes (conjunctival injection) (5) swollen lymph node in the neck of at least 15 millimeters.

Many children, especially infants, eventually diagnosed with Kawasaki disease do not exhibit all of the above criteria. In fact, many experts now recommend treating for Kawasaki disease even if only three days of fever have passed and at least three diagnostic criteria are present, especially if other tests reveal abnormalities consistent with Kawasaki disease. In addition, the diagnosis can be made purely by the detection of coronary artery aneurysms in the proper clinical setting.

Investigations

A physical examination will demonstrate many of the features listed above.

Blood tests

- Complete blood count (CBC) may reveal normocytic anemia and eventually thrombocytosis
- Erythrocyte sedimentation rate (ESR) will be elevated
- C-reactive protein (CRP) will be elevated
- Liver function tests may show evidence of hepatic inflammation and low serum albumin

Other optional tests

- Electrocardiogram may show evidence of ventricular dysfunction or, occasionally, arrhythmia due to myocarditis
- Echocardiogram may show subtle coronary artery changes or, later, true aneurysms.
- Ultrasound or computerized tomography may show hydrops (enlargement) of the gallbladder
- Urinalysis may show white blood cells and protein in the urine (pyuria and proteinuria) without evidence of bacterial growth
- Lumbar puncture may show evidence of aseptic meningitis
- Angiography was historically used to detect coronary artery aneurysms and remains the gold standard for their detection, but is rarely used today unless coronary artery aneurysms have already been detected by echocardiography.

Treatment

Children with Kawasaki disease should be hospitalized and cared for by a physician who has experience with this disease. When in an academic medical center, care is often shared between pediatric cardiology and pediatric infectious disease specialists (although no specific infectious agent has been identified yet).[13] It is imperative that treatment be started as soon as the diagnosis is made to prevent damage to the coronary arteries.

Intravenous immunoglobulin (IVIG) is the standard treatment for Kawasaki disease[22] and is administered in high doses with marked improvement usually noted within 24 hours. If the fever does not respond, an additional dose may have to be considered. In rare cases, a third dose may be given to the child. IVIG by itself is most useful within the first seven days of onset of fever, in terms of preventing coronary artery aneurysm.

Salicylate therapy, particularly aspirin, remains an important part of the treatment (though questioned by some)[23] but salicylates alone are not as effective as Intravenous immunoglobulin. Aspirin therapy is started at high doses until the fever subsides, and then is continued at a low dose when the patient returns home, usually for two months to prevent blood clots from forming. Except for Kawasaki disease and a few other indications, aspirin is otherwise normally not recommended for children due to its association with Reye's syndrome. Because childern with kawasaki disease will be taking aspirin for up to several months, vaccination against varicella and influenza is required, as these infections are most likely to cause Reyes syndrome.[24]

Corticosteroids have also been used,[25] especially when other treatments fail or symptoms recur, but in a randomized controlled trial, the addition of corticosteroid to immune globulin and aspirin did not improve outcome. [26] In cases of kawasaki disease refractory to intravenous immunoglobulin, cyclophosphamide and plasma exchange has been investigated as a possible treatments with varible results.[27]

There are also treatments for iritis and other eye symptoms. Other treatment may include the use of Infliximab (Remicade). Infliximab works by binding tumour necrosis factor alpha.

Epidemiology

By far the highest incidence of Kawasaki disease occurs in Japan (175 per 100,000), though its incidence in the United States is increasing. Kawasaki disease is predominantly a disease of young children, with 80% of patients younger than five years of age. The disease affects boys more than girls. Kawasaki was extremely uncommon in caucasians until the last few decades. Approximately 2,000-4,000 cases are identified in the United States each year.[12] [13]

Prognosis

With early treatment, rapid recovery from the acute symptoms can be expected and the risk of coronary artery aneurysms greatly reduced. Untreated, the acute symptoms of Kawasaki disease are self-limited (*i.e.* the patient will recover eventually), but the risk of coronary artery involvement is much greater. Overall, about 2% of patients die from complications of coronary vasculitis. Patients who have had Kawasaki disease should have an echocardiogram initially every few weeks, and then every one or two years to screen for progression of cardiac involvement.

It is also not uncommon that a relapse of symptoms may occur soon after initial treatment with IVIG. This usually requires re-hospitalization and re-treatment. Treatment with IVIG can cause allergic and non-allergic acute reactions, aseptic meningitis, fluid overload and, rarely, other serious reactions. Overall, life-threatening complications resulting from therapy for Kawasaki disease are exceedingly rare, especially compared with the risk of non-treatment.

See also

- List of cutaneous conditions

External links

- Kawasaki Disease Foundation [28]
- Kawasaki Disease Canada [29]
- Kawasaki Disease Forum [30]
- Kawasaki Disease Research Program [31]
- Kawasaki Disease information [32] from Seattle Children's Hospital Heart Center
- Kawasaki Disease [33], MedlinePlus
- Australian Kawasaki Support Network [34]
- Kawasaki Disease Foundation of South Africa [35]

References

[1] http://apps.who.int/classifications/apps/icd/icd10online/?gm30.htm+m303
[2] http://www.icd9data.com/getICD9Code.ashx?icd9=446.1
[3] http://www.ncbi.nlm.nih.gov/entrez/dispomim.cgi?id=611775
[4] http://www.diseasesdatabase.com/ddb7121.htm
[5] http://www.nlm.nih.gov/medlineplus/ency/article/000989.htm
[6] http://www.emedicine.com/ped/topic1236.htm
[7] http://www.nlm.nih.gov/cgi/mesh/2009/MB_cgi?field=uid&term=D009080
[8] Rapini, Ronald P.; Bolognia, Jean L.; Jorizzo, Joseph L. (2007). *Dermatology: 2-Volume Set*. St. Louis: Mosby. pp. 1232-4. ISBN 1-4160-2999-0.
[9] Merck Manual, (http://www.merck.com/mmpe/print/sec19/ch286/ch286c.html) Online edition, Kawasaki Disease]
[10] Kawasaki T (1967). "[Acute febrile mucocutaneous syndrome with lymphoid involvement with specific desquamation of the fingers and toes in children]" (in Japanese). *Arerugi* **16** (3): 178–222. PMID 6062087 (http://www.ncbi.nlm.nih.gov/pubmed/6062087).
[11] Park AH, Batchra N, Rowley A, Hotaling A (May 1997). "Patterns of Kawasaki syndrome presentation" (http://linkinghub.elsevier.com/retrieve/pii/S0165587697014948). *Int. J. Pediatr. Otorhinolaryngol.* **40** (1): 41–50. doi: 10.1016/S0165-5876(97)01494-8 (http://dx.doi.org/10.1016/S0165-5876(97)01494-8). PMID 9184977 (http://www.ncbi.nlm.nih.gov/pubmed/9184977). .
[12] "Kawasaki Disease - Signs and Symptoms" (http://www.ucsfhealth.org/childrens/medical_services/heart_center/acquired/conditions/kawasaki/signs.html). .
[13] "Who Kawasaki Disease Affects" (http://www.childrenshospital.org/clinicalservices/Site468/mainpageS468P5.html). Children's Hospital Boston. . Retrieved 2009-01-04.
[14] Rowley AH, Baker SC, Orenstein JM, Shulman ST (May 2008). "Searching for the cause of Kawasaki disease--cytoplasmic inclusion bodies provide new insight". *Nat. Rev. Microbiol.* **6** (5): 394–401. doi: 10.1038/nrmicro1853 (http://dx.doi.org/10.1038/nrmicro1853). PMID 18364728 (http://www.ncbi.nlm.nih.gov/pubmed/18364728).
[15] "Kawasaki Disease" (http://www.americanheart.org/presenter.jhtml?identifier=4634). American Heart Association. . Retrieved 3 January 2009.
[16] "Kawasaki Disease: Causes" (http://www.mayoclinic.com/health/kawasaki-disease/DS00576/DSECTION=causes). Mayo Clinic. . Retrieved 3 January 2009.
[17] Nakamura Y, Yashiro M, Uehara R, Oki I, Watanabe M, Yanagawa H (2008). "Monthly observation of the number of patients with Kawasaki disease and its incidence rates in Japan: chronological and geographical observation from nationwide surveys" (http://joi.jlc.jst.go.jp/JST.JSTAGE/jea/JE2008030?from=PubMed) (– [Scholar search] (http://scholar.google.co.uk/scholar?hl=en&lr=&q=intitle:Monthly+observation+of+the+number+of+patients+with+Kawasaki+disease+and+its+incidence+rates+in+Japan:+chronological+and+geographical+observation+from+nationwide+surveys&as_publication=J+Epidemiol&as_ylo=2008&as_yhi=2008&btnG=Search)). *J Epidemiol* **18** (6): 273–9. doi: 10.2188/jea.JE2008030 (http://dx.doi.org/10.2188/jea.JE2008030). PMID 19075496 (http://www.ncbi.nlm.nih.gov/pubmed/19075496). .
[18] Freeman AF, Shulman ST (June 2001). "Recent developments in Kawasaki disease". *Curr Opin Infect Dis* **14** (3): 357–61. PMID 11964855 (http://www.ncbi.nlm.nih.gov/pubmed/11964855).
[19] Onouchi Y, Gunji T, Burns JC, *et al.* (January 2008). "ITPKC functional polymorphism associated with Kawasaki disease susceptibility and formation of coronary artery aneurysms". *Nat. Genet.* **40** (1): 35–42. doi: 10.1038/ng.2007.59 (http://dx.doi.org/10.1038/ng.2007.59). PMID 18084290 (http://www.ncbi.nlm.nih.gov/pubmed/18084290).
[20] Keren G, Danon YL, Orgad S, Kalt R, Gazit E (August 1982). "HLA Bw51 is increased in mucocutaneous lymph node syndrome in Israeli patients". *Tissue Antigens* **20** (2): 144–6. PMID 6958087 (http://www.ncbi.nlm.nih.gov/pubmed/6958087).
[21] "Kawasaki Disease - June 1999 - American Academy of Family Physicians" (http://www.aafp.org/afp/990600ap/3093.html). .
[22] Oates-Whitehead RM, Baumer JH, Haines L, *et al.* (2003). "Intravenous immunoglobulin for the treatment of Kawasaki disease in children". *Cochrane Database Syst Rev* (4): CD004000. doi: 10.1002/14651858.CD004000 (http://dx.doi.org/10.1002/14651858.CD004000). PMID 14584002 (http://www.ncbi.nlm.nih.gov/pubmed/14584002).
[23] Hsieh KS, Weng KP, Lin CC, Huang TC, Lee CL, Huang SM (December 2004). "Treatment of acute Kawasaki disease: aspirin's role in the febrile stage revisited" (http://pediatrics.aappublications.org/cgi/pmidlookup?view=long&pmid=15545617). *Pediatrics* **114** (6): e689–93. doi: 10.1542/peds.2004-1037 (http://dx.doi.org/10.1542/peds.2004-1037). PMID 15545617 (http://www.ncbi.nlm.nih.gov/pubmed/15545617). .
[24] http://emedicine.medscape.com/article/804960-treatment
[25] Sundel RP, Baker AL, Fulton DR, Newburger JW (June 2003). "Corticosteroids in the initial treatment of Kawasaki disease: report of a randomized trial" (http://linkinghub.elsevier.com/retrieve/pii/S0022347603001173). *J. Pediatr.* **142** (6): 611–6. doi: 10.1067/mpd.2003.191 (http://dx.doi.org/10.1067/mpd.2003.191). PMID 12838187 (http://www.ncbi.nlm.nih.gov/pubmed/12838187). .
[26] Newburger JW et al., Randomized trial of pulsed corticosteroid therapy for primary treatment of Kawasaki disease, N Engl J Med. 2007 Feb 25;356(7):663-75
[27] http://www.emedicine.medscape.com/article/804960-treatment
[28] http://www.kdfoundation.org/

[29] http://www.kdcanada.ca/
[30] http://www.kdforum.org/
[31] http://www.emory.edu/CHCS/p_histmed_Kawasaki.ht
[32] http://heart.seattlechildrens.org/conditions_treated/kawasaki_disease.asp
[33] http://www.nlm.nih.gov/medlineplus/kawasakidisease.html
[34] http://www.kdfoundation.org.au/
[35] http://www.kawasakidiseasefoundation.co.za/

Skin

The **skin** is a soft outer covering of an animal, in particular a vertebrate. Other animal coverings such the arthropod exoskeleton or the seashell has different developmental origin, structure and chemical composition. The adjective **cutaneous** literally means "of the skin" (from Latin *cutis*, skin). In mammals, the skin is the largest organ of the integumentary system made up of multiple layers of ectodermal tissue, and guards the underlying muscles, bones, ligaments and internal organs.[1] Skin of a different nature exists in amphibians, reptiles, birds.[2] All mammals have some hair on their skin, even marine mammals which appear to be hairless. Because it interfaces with the environment, skin plays a key role in protecting (the body) against pathogens[3] and excessive water loss.[4] Its other functions are insulation, temperature regulation, sensation, and the protection of vitamin B folates. Severely damaged skin will try to heal by forming scar tissue. This is often discolored and depigmented.

Hair with sufficient density is called fur. The fur mainly serves to augment the insulation the skin provides, but can also serve as a secondary sexual characteristic or as camouflage. On some animals, the skin is very hard and thick, and can be processed to create leather. Reptiles and fish have hard protective scales on their skin for protection, and birds have hard feathers, all made of tough β-keratins. Amphibian skin is not a strong barrier to passage of chemicals and is often subject to osmosis. A frog sitting in an anesthetic solution could quickly go to sleep.

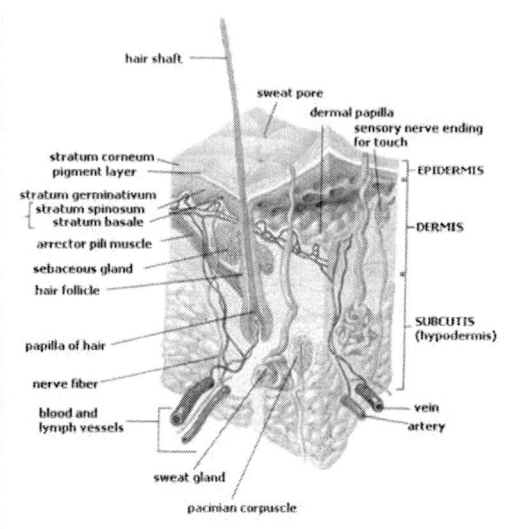

Layers of mammal skin: epidermis, dermis, and subcutis, showing a hair follicle, sweat gland & sebaceous gland.

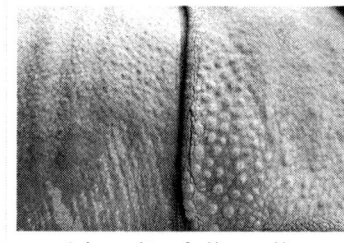

A close up picture of a rhinoceros skin.

Functions

Skin performs the following functions:

1. Protection: an anatomical barrier from pathogens and damage between the internal and external environment in bodily defense; Langerhans cells in the skin are part of the adaptive immune system.[3] [4]
2. Sensation: contains a variety of nerve endings that react to heat and cold, touch, pressure, vibration, and tissue injury; see somatosensory system and haptics.
3. Heat regulation: the skin contains a blood supply far greater than its requirements which allows precise control of energy loss by radiation, convection and conduction. Dilated blood vessels increase perfusion and heatloss, while constricted vessels greatly reduce cutaneous blood flow and conserve heat. Erector pili muscles are significant in animals.
4. Control of evaporation: the skin provides a relatively dry and semi-impermeable barrier to fluid loss.[4]
5. Storage and synthesis: acts as a storage center for lipids and water
6. Absorption: Oxygen, nitrogen and carbon dioxide can diffuse into the epidermis in small amounts, some animals using their skin for their sole respiration organ (contrary to popular belief, however, humans do not absorb oxygen through the skin).[5]
7. Water resistance: The skin acts as a water resistant barrier so essential nutrients aren't washed out of the body.

Animal skin products

The term skin refers to the covering of a small animal, such as a sheep, goat (goatskin), pig, snake (snakeskin) etc or the young of a large animal.

The term hides or rawhide refers to the covering of a large adult animal such as a cow, buffalo, horse etc.

Skins and hides from different animals are used for clothing, bags and other consumer products, usually in the form of leather, but also furs.

Skin can also be cooked to make pork rind or cracklin. The skin on roasted chicken and turkey is another coveted delicacy.

Mammalian skin layers

Mammalian skin is composed of three primary layers:

- the *epidermis*, which provides waterproofing and serves as a barrier to infection;
- the *dermis*, which serves as a location for the appendages of skin; and
- the *hypodermis (subcutaneous adipose layer)*.

Epidermis

Epidermis, "epi" coming from the Greek meaning "over" or "upon", is the outermost layer of the skin. It forms the waterproof, protective wrap over the body's surface and is made up of stratified squamous epithelium with an underlying basal lamina.

The epidermis contains no blood vessels, and cells in the deepest layers are nourished by diffusion from blood capillaries extending to the upper layers of the dermis. The main type of cells which make up the epidermis are Merkel cells, keratinocytes, with melanocytes and Langerhans cells also present. The epidermis can be further subdivided into the following *strata* (beginning with the outermost layer): corneum, lucidum (only in palms of hands and bottoms of feet), granulosum, spinosum, basale. Cells are formed through mitosis at the basale layer. The daughter cells (see cell division) move up the strata changing shape and composition as they die due to isolation from their blood source. The cytoplasm is released and the protein keratin is inserted. They eventually reach the corneum and slough off (desquamation). This process is called *keratinization* and takes place within about 27 days.

This keratinized layer of skin is responsible for keeping water in the body and keeping other harmful chemicals and pathogens out, making skin a natural barrier to infection.

Components

The epidermis contains no blood vessels, and is nourished by diffusion from the dermis. The main type of cells which make up the epidermis are keratinocytes, melanocytes, Langerhans cells and Merkels cells. The epidermis helps the skin to regulate body temperature.

Layers

Epidermis is divided into several layers where cells are formed through mitosis at the innermost layers. They move up the strata changing shape and composition as they differentiate and become filled with keratin. They eventually reach the top layer called *stratum corneum* and are sloughed off, or desquamated. This process is called *keratinization* and takes place within weeks. The outermost layer of the epidermis consists of 25 to 30 layers of dead cells.

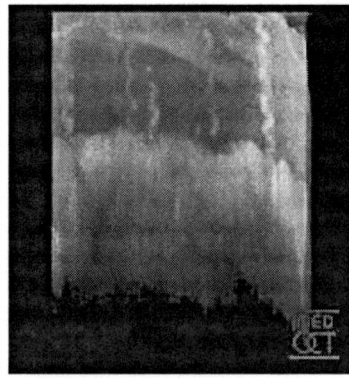

[*also see: image rotating (1.1 mb)*]
Optical Coherence Tomography tomogram of fingertip, depicting stratum corneum (~500 μm thick) with stratum disjunctum on top and stratum lucidum (connection to stratum spinosum) in the middle. At the bottom superficial parts of the dermis. Sweatducts are clearly visible.

Sublayers

Epidermis is divided into the following 5 sublayers or strata:

- Stratum corneum
- Stratum lucidum
- Stratum granulosum
- Stratum spinosum
- Stratum germinativum (also called "stratum basale")

Mnemonics that are good for remembering the layers of the skin (using "stratum basale" instead of "stratum germinativum"):

- "**C**her **L**ikes **G**etting **S**kin **B**otoxed" (from superficial to deep)
- "**B**efore **S**igning, **G**et **L**egal **C**ounsel" (from deep to superficial)

Blood capillaries are found beneath the epidermis, and are linked to an arteriole and a venule. Arterial shunt vessels may bypass the network in ears, the nose and fingertips.

Dermis
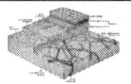
The distribution of the bloodvessels in the skin of the sole of the foot. (Corium - TA alternate term for dermis - is labeled at upper right.)
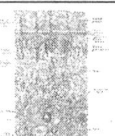

A diagrammatic sectional view of the skin (*click on image to magnify*). (Dermis labeled at center right.)	
Gray's	*subject #234 1065* [6]
MeSH	*Dermis* [7]
Dorlands/Elsevier	*Skin* [8]

Dermis

The **dermis** is the layer of skin beneath the epidermis that consists of connective tissue and cushions the body from stress and strain. The dermis is tightly connected to the epidermis by a basement membrane. It also harbors many Mechanoreceptors (nerve endings) that provide the sense of touch and heat. It contains the hair follicles, sweat glands, sebaceous glands, apocrine glands, lymphatic vessels and blood vessels. The blood vessels in the dermis provide nourishment and waste removal from its own cells as well as from the Stratum basale of the epidermis.

The dermis is structurally divided into two areas: a superficial area adjacent to the epidermis, called the *papillary region*, and a deep thicker area known as the *reticular region*.

Papillary region

The papillary region is composed of loose areolar connective tissue. It is named for its fingerlike projections called *papillae*, that extend toward the epidermis. The papillae provide the dermis with a "bumpy" surface that interdigitates with the epidermis, strengthening the connection between the two layers of skin.

Reticular region

The reticular region lies deep in the papillary region and is usually much thicker. It is composed of dense irregular connective tissue, and receives its name from the dense concentration of collagenous, elastic, and reticular fibers that weave throughout it. These protein fibers give the dermis its properties of strength, extensibility, and elasticity.

Also located within the reticular region are the roots of the hair, sebaceous glands, sweat glands, receptors, nails, and blood vessels.

Hypodermis

The hypodermis is not part of the skin, and lies below the dermis. Its purpose is to attach the skin to underlying bone and muscle as well as supplying it with blood vessels and nerves. It consists of loose connective tissue and elastin. The main cell types are fibroblasts, macrophages and adipocytes (the hypodermis contains 50% of body fat). Fat serves as padding and insulation for the body. Another name for the hypodermis is the subcutaneous tissue.

Microorganisms like *Staphylococcus epidermidis* colonize the skin surface. The density of skin flora depends on region of the skin. The disinfected skin surface gets recolonized from bacteria residing in the deeper areas of the hair follicle, gut and urogenital openings.

In fish and amphibians

The epidermis of fish and of most amphibians consists entirely of live cells, with only minimal quantities of keratin in the cells of the superficial layer. It is generally permeable, and, in the case of many amphibians, may actually be a major respiratory organ. The dermis of bony fish typically contains relatively little of the connective tissue found in tetrapods. Instead, in most species, it is largely replaced by solid, protective bony scales. Apart from some particularly large dermal bones that form parts of the skull, these scales are lost in tetrapods, although many reptiles do have scales of a different kind, as do pangolins. Cartilaginous fish have numerous tooth-like denticles embedded in their skin, in place of true scales.

Sweat glands and sebaceous glands are both unique to mammals, but other types of skin gland are found in other vertebrates. Fish typically have a numerous individual mucus-secreting skin cells that aid in insulation and protection, but may also have poison glands, photophores, or cells that produce a more watery, serous fluid. In amphibians, the mucus cells are gathered together to form sac-like glands. Most living amphibians also possess *granular glands* in the skin, that secrete irritating or toxic compounds.[9]

Although melanin is found in the skin of many species, in reptiles, amphibians, and fish, the epidermis is often relatively colourless. Instead, the colour of the skin is largely due to chromatophores in the dermis, which, in addition to melanin, may contain guanine or carotenoid pigments. Many species, such as chameleons and flounders may be able to change the colour of their skin by adjusting the relative size of their chromatophores.[9]

In birds and reptiles

The epidermis of birds and reptiles is closer to that of mammals, with a layer of dead keratin-filled cells at the surface, to help reduce water loss. A similar pattern is also seen in some of the more terrestrial amphibians, such as toads. However, in all of these animals there is no clear differentiation of the epidermis into distinct layers, as occurs in humans, with the change in cell type being relatively gradual. The mammalian epidermis always possesses at least a stratum germinativum and stratum corneum, but the other intermediate layers found in humans are not always distinguishable. Hair is a distinctive feature of mammalian skin, while feathers are (at least among living species) similarly unique to birds.[9]

Birds and reptiles have relatively few skin glands, although there may be a few structures for specific purposes, such as pheromone-secreting cells in some reptiles, or the uropygial gland of most birds.[9]

See also

- Acid mantle
- Callus - thick area of skin
- Cutaneous structure development
- Hair - including hair follicles in skin
- Intertriginous
- Moult
- Meissner's corpuscle
- Pacinian corpuscle
- Rawhide
- Superficial fascia

References

[1] "Skin care" (analysis), Health-Cares.net, 2007, webpage: HCcare (http://skin-care.health-cares.net/oily-skin-care.php).
[2] Alibardi L. (2003). Adaptation to the land: The skin of reptiles in comparison to that of amphibians and endotherm amniotes. J Exp Zoolog B Mol Dev Evol. 298(1):12-41. PMID 12949767
[3] Proksch E, Brandner JM, Jensen JM. (2008).The skin: an indispensable barrier. Exp Dermatol. 17(12):1063-72. PMID 19043850
[4] Madison KC. (2003). Barrier function of the skin: "la raison d'être" of the epidermis (http://www.nature.com/jid/journal/v121/n2/pdf/5601872a.pdf). J Invest Dermatol. 121(2):231-41. PMID 12880413
[5] Connor, Steven: *The book of skin*, Cornell University Press, 2003, pg. 176
[6] http://education.yahoo.com/reference/gray/subjects/subject?id=234#p1065
[7] http://www.nlm.nih.gov/cgi/mesh/2007/MB_cgi?mode=&term=Dermis
[8] http://www.mercksource.com/pp/us/cns/cns_hl_dorlands_split.jsp?pg=/ppdocs/us/common/dorlands/dorland/seven/000097765.htm
[9] Romer, Alfred Sherwood; Parsons, Thomas S. (1977). *The Vertebrate Body*. Philadelphia, PA: Holt-Saunders International. pp. 129–145. ISBN 0-03-910284-X.

Mucous membrane

Mucous membrane
Serosa / Longitudinal Muscle / Myenteric Plexus / Circular Muscle / Submucosal Plexus / Submucosal / Mucosal
LAYERS: serosa / longitudinal muscle / myenteric plexus / circular muscle / submucosal plexus / submucosal / mucosal
Section of the human esophagus. Moderately magnified. The section is transverse and from near the middle of the gullet. a. Fibrous covering. b. Divided fibers of longitudinal muscular coat. c. Transverse muscular fibers. d. Submucous or **areolar** layer. e. Muscularis mucosae. f. Mucous membrane, with vessels and part of a lymphoid nodule. g. Stratified epithelial lining. h. Mucous gland. i. Gland duct. m'. Striated muscular fibers cut across.

Latin	*tunica mucosa*
Gray's	*subject #242 1110* [1]
Dorlands/Elsevier	*Mucous membrane* [2]

The **mucous membranes** (or **mucosae**; singular **mucosa**) are linings of mostly endodermal origin, covered in epithelium, which are involved in absorption and secretion. They line various body cavities that are exposed to the external environment and internal organs. It is at several places continuous with skin: at the nostrils, the lips, the ears, the genital area, and the anus. The sticky, thick fluid secreted by the mucous membranes and gland is termed mucus. The term *mucous membrane* refers to where they are found in the body and not every mucous membrane secretes mucus.

Body cavities featuring mucous membrane include most of the respiratory system. The glans penis (head of the penis) and glans clitoridis, along with the inside of the prepuce (foreskin) and the clitoral hood, are mucous membranes. The urethra is also a mucous membrane. The secreted mucus traps the pathogens in the body, preventing any further activities of diseases.

Components

- Epithelium
- Lamina propria
- Smooth muscle/Muscularis mucosa/ (GI tract)

Some examples of mucosa

- Buccal mucosa
- Esophageal mucosa
- Gastric mucosa
- Intestinal mucosa
- Nasal mucosa
- Olfactory mucosa
- Oral mucosa
- Bronchial mucosa
- Uterine mucosa
- Endometrium is the mucosa of the uterus
- Penile mucosa

Additional images

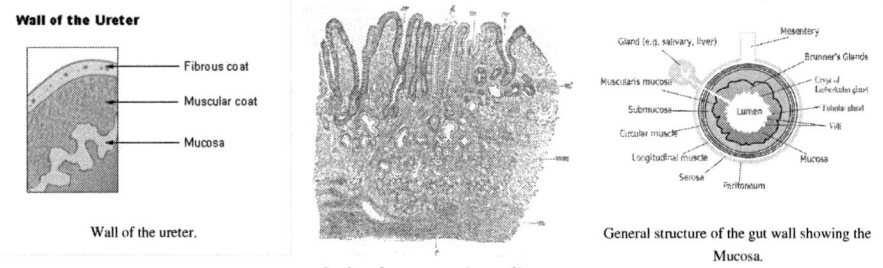

Wall of the ureter.

Section of mucous membrane of human stomach, near the cardiac orifice.

General structure of the gut wall showing the Mucosa.

Mucous membrane

See also
- Mucin
- Mucocutaneous boundary
- Mucociliary clearance
- Mucosal immune system

External links
- *mucosa* [3] at eMedicine Dictionary
- Organology at UC Davis *Digestive/mammal/system1/system4* [4] - "Mammal, whole system (LM, Low)"
- MeSH *Mucous+Membrane* [5]

References
[1] http://education.yahoo.com/reference/gray/subjects/subject?id=242#p1110
[2] http://www.mercksource.com/pp/us/cns/cns_hl_dorlands_split.jsp?pg=/ppdocs/us/common/dorlands/dorland/five/000064454.htm
[3] http://www.emedicinehealth.com/script/main/srchcont_dict.asp?src=mucosa
[4] http://trc.ucdavis.edu/mjguinan/apc100/modules/Digestive/mammal/system1/system4.html
[5] http://www.nlm.nih.gov/cgi/mesh/2009/MB_cgi?mode=&term=Mucous+Membrane

Lymph node

A **lymph node** (pronounced /'lɪmf noʊd/) is a small bean-shaped organ of the immune system, distributed widely throughout the body and linked by lymphatic vessels. Lymph nodes are garrisons of B, T, and other immune cells. Lymph nodes are found all through the body, and act as filters or traps for foreign particles. They contain white blood cells that use oxygen to process. Thus they are important in the proper functioning of the immune system.

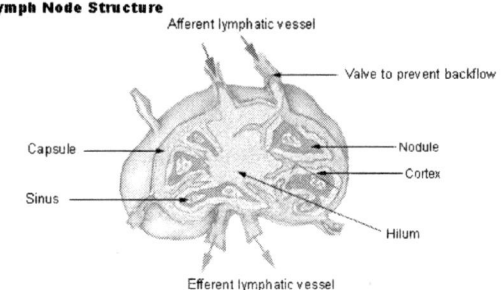

A lymph node showing afferent and efferent lymphatic vessels

Lymph nodes also have clinical significance. They become inflamed or enlarged in various conditions, which may range from trivial, such as a throat infection, to life-threatening such as cancers. In the latter, the condition of lymph nodes is so significant that it is used for cancer staging, which decides the treatment to be employed, and for determining the prognosis.

Lymph nodes can also be diagnosed by biopsy whenever they are inflamed. Certain diseases affect lymph nodes with characteristic consistency and location.

Function

Pathogens, or germs, can set up infections anywhere in the body. However, lymphocytes, a type of white blood cell, will meet the antigens, or proteins, in the peripheral lymphoid organs, which includes lymph nodes. The antigens are displayed by specialized cells in the lymph nodes. Naive lymphocytes (meaning the cells have not encountered an antigen yet) enter the node from the bloodstream, through specialized capillary venules. After the lymphocytes specialize they will exit the lymph node through the efferent lymphatic vessel with the rest of the lymph. The lymphocytes continuously recirculate the peripheral lymphoid organs and the state of the lymph nodes depends on infection. During an infection, the lymph nodes can expand due to intense B-cell proliferation in the germinal centers, a condition commonly referred to as "swollen glands".

Structure

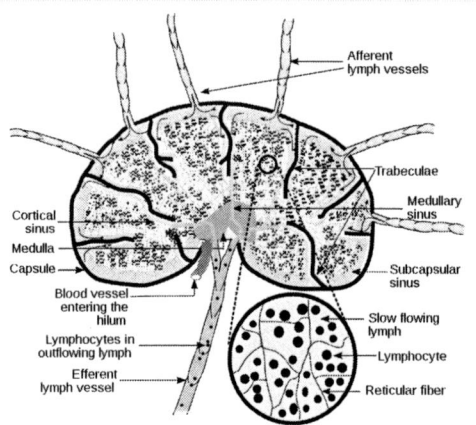

Schematic diagram of lymph node showing the flow of lymph through the lymph sinuses. Note: Outflowing lymph has more lymphocytes

The lymph node is surrounded by a fibrous capsule, and inside the lymph node the fibrous capsule extends to form trabeculae. The substance of the lymph node is divided into the outer cortex and the inner medulla surrounded by the former all around except for at the hilum, where the medulla comes in direct contact with the surface.[1]

Thin reticular fibers, elastin and reticular fibers form a supporting meshwork called *reticular network* (RN) inside the node, within which the white blood cells (WBCs), most prominently, lymphocytes are tightly packed as follicles in the cortex. Elsewhere, there are only occasional WBCs. The RN provides not just the structural support, but also provide surface for adhesion of the dendritic cells, macrophages and lymphocytes. It allows for exchange of material with blood through the high endothelial venules and provides the growth and regulatory factors necessary for activation and maturation of immune cells.[2]

The number and composition of follicles can change especially when challenged by an antigen, when they develop a germinal center.[1]

A lymph sinus is a channel within the lymph node lined by the endothelial cells along with fibroblastic reticular cells and allows for smooth flow of lymph through them. Thus, subcapsular sinus is a sinus immediately deep to the capsule, and its endothelium is continuous with that of the afferent lymph vessel. It is also continuous with similar sinuses flanking the trabeculae and within the cortex (cortical sinuses). The cortical sinuses and that flanking the trabeculae drain into the *medullary sinuses*, from where the lymph flows into the efferent lymph vessel.[1]

Multiple afferent lymph vessels that branch and network extensively within the capsule bring lymph into the lymph node. This lymph enters the subcapsular sinus. The innermost lining of the afferent lymph vessels is continuous with the cells lining the lymph sinuses.[1] The lymph gets slowly filtered through the substance of the lymph node and ultimately reaches the medulla. In its course it encounters the lymphocytes and may lead to their activation as a part of adaptive immune response.

The concave side of the lymph node is called the hilum. The efferent attaches to the hilum by a relatively dense reticulum present there, and carries the lymph out of the lymph node.

Cortex

In the cortex, the subcapsular sinus drains to *cortical sinuses*.

The outer cortex consists mainly of the B cells arranged as follicles, which may develop a germinal center when challenged with an antigen, and the deeper cortex mainly consisting of the T cells. There is a zone known as the subcortical zone where T-cells (or cells that are mainly red) mainly interact with dendritic cells, and where the reticular network is dense.[3]

Medulla

There are two named structures in the medulla:
- The *medullary cords* are cords of lymphatic tissue, and include plasma cells and B cells
- The *medullary sinuses* (or *sinusoids*) are vessel-like spaces separating the medullary cords. The Lymph flows into the medullary sinuses from cortical sinuses, and into efferent lymphatic vessels. Medullary sinuses contain histiocytes (immobile macrophages) and reticular cells.

Shape and size

Human lymph nodes are bean-shaped and range in size from a few millimeters to about 1–2 cm in their normal state.[1] They may become enlarged due to a tumor or infection. Lymphocytes, also known as white blood cells are located within honeycomb structures of the lymph nodes. Lymph nodes are enlarged when the body is infected, primarily because there is an elevated rate of trafficking of lymphocytes into the node from the blood, exceeding the rate of outflow from the node, and secondarily as a result of the activation and proliferation of antigen-specific T and B cells (clonal expansion). In some cases they may feel enlarged because of a previous infection; although one may be healthy, one may still feel them residually enlarged.

Lymphatic circulation

Lymph circulates to the lymph node via *afferent lymphatic vessels* and drains into the node just beneath the capsule in a space called the *subcapsular sinus*. The subcapsular sinus drains into trabecular sinuses and finally into medullary sinuses. The sinus space is criss-crossed by the pseudopods of macrophages which act to trap foreign particles and filter the lymph. The medullary sinuses converge at the hilum and lymph then leaves the lymph node via the *efferent lymphatic vessel* towards either a more central lymph node or ultimately for drainage into a central venous subclavian blood vessel, most via Virchow's node and Ductus thoracicus. Valves on the afferent side prevent backflow.

Lymphocytes, both B cells and T cells, constantly circulate through the lymph nodes. They enter the lymph node via the postcapillary venules, and cross its wall by the process of diapedesis.

- The B cells migrate to the nodular cortex and medulla.
- The T cells migrate to the deep cortex ("paracortex").

When a lymphocyte recognizes an antigen, B cells become activated and migrate to germinal centers (by definition, a "secondary nodule" has a germinal center, while a "primary nodule" does not). When antibody-producing plasma cells are formed, they migrate to the medullary cords. Stimulation of the lymphocytes by antigens can accelerate the migration process to about 10 times normal, resulting in characteristic swelling of the lymph nodes.

The spleen and tonsils are large lymphoid organs that serve similar functions to lymph nodes, though the spleen filters blood cells rather than lymph.

Distribution

Humans have approximately 500-600 lymph nodes distributed throughout the body, with clusters found in the underarms, groin, neck, chest, and abdomen.

Lymph nodes of the human head and neck

- Cervical lymph nodes
  - Anterior cervical: These nodes, both superficial and deep, lie above and beneath the sternocleidomastoid muscles. They drain the internal structures of the throat as well as part of the posterior pharynx, tonsils, and thyroid gland.
  - Posterior cervical: These nodes extend in a line posterior to the sternocleidomastoids but in front of the trapezius, from the level of the Mastoid portion of the temporal bone to the clavicle. They are frequently enlarged during upper respiratory infections.
- Tonsillar (sub mandibular): These nodes are located just below the angle of the mandible. They drain the tonsillar and posterior pharyngeal regions.
- Sub-mandibular: These nodes run along the underside of the jaw on either side. They drain the structures in the floor of the mouth.
- Sub-mental: These nodes are just below the chin. They drain the teeth and intra-oral cavity.
- Supraclavicular lymph nodes: These nodes are in the hollow above the clavicle, just lateral to where it joins the sternum. They drain a part of the thoracic cavity and abdomen. Virchow's node is a left supraclavicular lymph node which receives the lymph drainage from most of the body (especially the abdomen) via the thoracic duct and is thus an early site of metastasis for various malignancies.

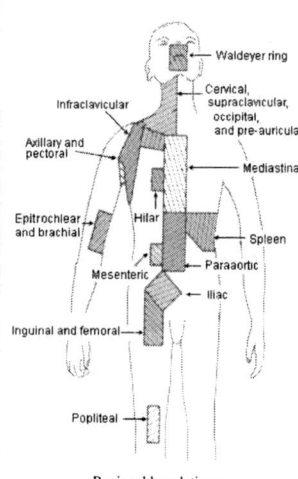

Regional lymph tissue

Lymph nodes of the thorax

- Lymph nodes of the lungs: The lymph is drained from the lung tissue through **subsegmental**, **segmental**, **lobar** and **interlobar** lymph nodes to the **hilar** lymph nodes, which are located around the hilum (the pedicle, which attaches the lung to the mediastinal structures, containing the pulmonary artery, the pulmonary veins, the main bronchus for each side, some vegetative nerves and the lymphatics) of each lung. The lymph flows subsequently to the mediastinal lymph nodes.
- Mediastinal lymph nodes: They consist of several lymp node groups, especially along the trachea (5 groups), along the esophagus and between the lung and the diaphragm. In the mediastinal lymph nodes arises lymphatic ducts, which draines the lymph to the left subclavian vein (to the venous angle in the confluence of the subclavian and deep jugular veins).

The mediastinal lymph nodes along the esophagus are in tight connection with the abdominal lymph nodes along the esophagus and the stomach. That fact facilitates spreading of tumors cells through these lymphatics in cases of cancers of the stomach and particularly of the esophagus. Through the mediastinum, the main lymphatic drainage from the abdominal organs goes via the thoracic duct (*ductus thoracicus*), which drains majority of the lymph from the abdomen to the above mentioned left venous angle.

Lymph nodes of the arm

These drain the whole of the arm, and are divided into two groups, superficial and deep. The superficial nodes are supplied by lymphatics which are present throughout the arm, but are particularly rich on the palm and flexor aspects of the digits.

- Superficial lymph glands of the arm:
  - Supratrochlear glands: Situated above the medial epicondyle of the humerus, medial to the basilic vein, they drain the C7 and C8 dermatomes.
  - Deltoideopectoral glands: Situated between the pectoralis major and deltoid muscles inferior to the clavicle.
- Deep lymph glands of the arm: These comprise the axillary glands, which are 20-30 individual glands and can be subdivided into:
  - Lateral glands
  - Anterior or pectoral glands
  - Posterior or subscapular glands
  - Central or intermediate glands
  - Medial or subclavicular glands

Lower limbs

- Superficial inguinal lymph nodes
- Deep inguinal lymph nodes

Pathology

Lymphadenopathy is a term meaning "disease of the lymph nodes." It is, however, almost synonymously used with "swollen / enlarged lymph nodes." In this case, the lymph nodes are palpable, and is a sign of various infections and diseases.

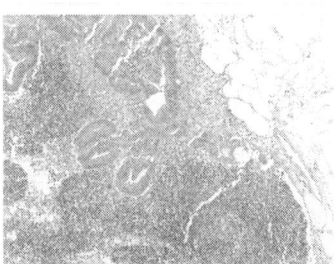

Micrograph of a mesenteric **lymph node** with colorectal adenocarcinoma, the most common type of colorectal cancer.

Lymph node

Additional images

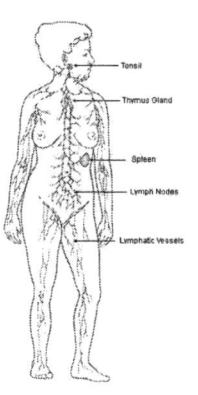
Lymphatic system

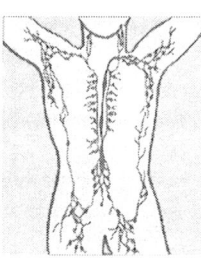
The human lymphatic system

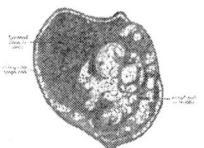
Section of small lymph node of rabbit. X 100.

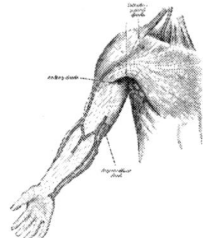
Lymphatics of the arm

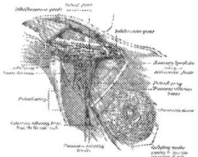
Lymphatics of the axillary region

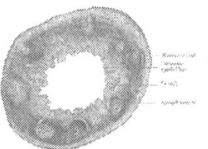
Transverse section of human vermiform process. X 20.

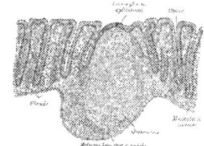
Section of mucous membrane of human rectum. X 60.

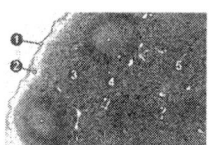
Lymph node, showing (1) capsule, (2) subscapular sinus, (3) germinal centers, (4) lymphoid nodule, (5?) HEVs.

See also

- Adenitis
- List of hæmatological diseases and malignancies
- Lymphadenectomy
- Lymphoma
- Histology at BU *07101loa* [4]

References

[1] Warwick, Roger; Peter L. Williams (1973) [1858]. "Angiology (Chapter 6)". *Gray's anatomy*. illustrated by Richard E. M. Moore (Thirty-fifth ed.). London: Longman. pp. 588–785.

[2] Kaldjian, Eric P.; J. Elizabeth Gretz, Arthur O. Anderson, Yinghui Shi and Stephen Shaw (October 2001). "Spatial and molecular organization of lymph node T cell cortex: a labyrinthine cavity bounded by an epithelium-like monolayer of fibroblastic reticular cells anchored to basement membrane-like extracellular matrix" (http://intimm.oxfordjournals.org/cgi/content/full/13/10/1243). *International Immunology* (Oxford Journals) **13** (10): 1243–1253. doi: 10.1093/intimm/13.10.1243 (http://dx.doi.org/10.1093/intimm/13.10.1243). . Retrieved 2008-07-11.

[3] Katakai, Tomoya; Takahiro Hara, Hiroyuki Gonda1, Manabu Sugai and Akira Shimizu (2004-07-05). "A novel reticular stromal structure in lymph node cortex: an immuno-platform for interactions among dendritic cells, T cells and B cells" (http://intimm.oxfordjournals.org/cgi/content/full/16/8/1133). *International Immunology* **16** (8): 1133–1142. doi: 10.1093/intimm/dxh113 (http://dx.doi.org/10.1093/intimm/dxh113). . Retrieved 2008-07-11.

[4] http://www.bu.edu/histology/p/07101loa.htm

Blood vessel

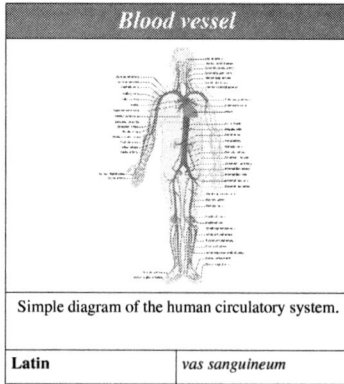

Simple diagram of the human circulatory system.

Latin	vas sanguineum

The **blood vessels** are the part of the circulatory system that transport blood throughout the body. There are three major types of blood vessels: the arteries, which carry the blood away from the heart, the capillaries, which enable the actual exchange of water and chemicals between the blood and the tissues; and the veins, which carry blood from the capillaries back towards the heart.

Anatomy

The arteries and veins have the same structure with three layers, from inside to outside.

- *Tunica intima* (the thinnest layer): a single layer of simple squamous endothelial cells glued by a polysaccharide intercellular matrix, surrounded by a thin layer of subendothelial connective tissue interlaced with a number of circularly arranged elastic bands called the *internal elastic lamina*.
- *Tunica media* (the thickest layer): circularly arranged elastic fiber, connective tissue, polysaccharide substances, the second and third layer are separated by another thick elastic band called external elastic lamina. The tunica media may (especially in arteries) be rich in vascular smooth muscle, which controls the caliber of the vessel.
- *Tunica adventitia*: entirely made of connective tissue. It also contains nerves that supply the vessel

as well as nutrient capillaries (vasa vasorum) in the larger blood vessels.

Capillaries consist of little more than a layer of endothelium and occasional connective tissue.

When blood vessels connect to form a region of diffuse vascular supply it is called an anastomosis (pl. anastomoses). Anastomoses provide critical alternative routes for blood to flow in case of blockages.

Laid end to end, all the blood vessels in an average human body would encircle the earth twice, a distance of approximately 100,000 kilometers.(60,000 miles)[1]

Types

There are various kinds of blood vessels:

- Arteries
  - Aorta (the largest artery, carries blood out of the heart)
  - Branches of the aorta, such as the carotid artery, the subclavian artery, the celiac trunk, the mesenteric arteries, the renal artery and the iliac artery.
- Arterioles
- Capillaries (the smallest blood vessels)
- Venules
- Veins
  - Large collecting vessels, such as the subclavian vein, the jugular vein, the renal vein and the iliac vein.
  - Venae cavae (the 2 largest veins, carry blood into the heart)

They are roughly grouped as *arterial* and *venous*, determined by whether the blood in it is flowing *away from* (arterial) or *toward* (venous) the heart. The term "arterial blood" is nevertheless used to indicate blood high in oxygen, although the pulmonary artery carries "venous blood" and blood flowing in the pulmonary vein is rich in oxygen. This is because they are carrying the blood to and from the lungs, respectively, to be oxygenated.

Physiology

Blood vessels do not actively engage in the transport of blood (they have no appreciable peristalsis), but arteries - and veins to a degree - can regulate their inner diameter by contraction of the muscular layer. This changes the blood flow to downstream organs, and is determined by the autonomic nervous system. Vasodilation and vasoconstriction are also used antagonistically as methods of thermoregulation.

Oxygen (bound to hemoglobin in red blood cells) is the most critical nutrient carried by the blood. In all arteries apart from the pulmonary artery, hemoglobin is highly saturated (95-100%) with oxygen. In all veins apart from the pulmonary vein, the hemoglobin is desaturated at about 75%. (The values are reversed in the pulmonary circulation.)

The blood pressure in blood vessels is traditionally expressed in millimetres of mercury (1 mmHg = 133 Pa). In the arterial system, this is usually around 120 mmHg systolic (high pressure wave due to contraction of the heart) and 80 mmHg diastolic (low pressure wave). In contrast, pressures in the venous system are constant and rarely exceed 10 mmHg.

Vasoconstriction is the constriction of blood vessels (narrowing, becoming smaller in cross-sectional area) by contracting the vascular smooth muscle in the vessel walls. It is regulated by vasoconstrictors (agents that cause vasoconstriction). These include paracrine factors (e.g. prostaglandins), a number of hormones (e.g. vasopressin and angiotensin) and neurotransmitters (e.g. epinephrine) from the nervous system.

Vasodilation is a similar process mediated by antagonistically acting mediators. The most prominent vasodilator is nitric oxide (termed endothelium-derived relaxing factor for this reason).

Permeability of the endothelium is pivotal in the release of nutrients to the tissue. It is also increased in inflammation in response to histamine, prostaglandins and interleukins, which leads to most of the symptoms of inflammation (swelling, redness and warmth).

Role in disease

Blood vessels play a role in virtually every medical condition. Cancer, for example, cannot progress unless the tumor causes angiogenesis (formation of new blood vessels) to supply the malignant cells' metabolic demand. Atherosclerosis, the formation of lipid lumps (atheromas) in the blood vessel wall, is the most common cardiovascular disease, the main cause of death in the Western world.

Blood vessel permeability is increased in inflammation. Damage, due to trauma or spontaneously, may lead to haemorrhage due to mechanical damage to the vessel endothelium. In contrast, occlusion of the blood vessel by atherosclerotic plaque, by an embolised blood clot or a foreign body leads to downstream ischemia (insufficient blood supply) and possibly necrosis. Vessel occlusion tends to be a positive feedback system; an occluded vessel creates eddies in the normally laminar flow or plug flow blood currents. These eddies create abnormal fluid velocity gradients which push blood elements such as cholesterol or chylomicron bodies to the endothelium. These deposit onto the arterial walls which are already partially occluded and build upon the blockage.[2]

Vasculitis is inflammation of the vessel wall, due to autoimmune disease or infection.

References

[1] "Heart, How it Works", American Heart Association (http://www.heartsource.org/presenter.jhtml?identifier=4642)
[2] Multiphase Flow and Fluidization, Gidaspow et al., Academic Press, 1992

Tomisaku Kawasaki

Tomisaku Kawasaki (Born 1925) is a Japanese pediatrician.[1]

Kawasaki disease is named for him. He published a description in Japanese in 1967, and a description in English in 1974.[2] [3] [4]

He first observed the condition in 1961.[5]

He studied at Chiba University. In Japan, there were several activities of etiology research groups, but there has been no established theory. He has been active in this field, and established "Japan Kawasaki Disease Research Center" in 1990 and later a non-profit organization "Japan Disease Research Center".From "Clinicians' Battles, Doctors whose names are found in the disease, (2000), edit. Itakura E. Medical Sense, Tokyo, in Japanese.

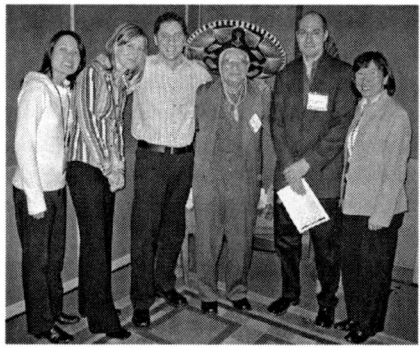

Dr. Tomisaku Kawasaki (centre right) at the 8th International Kawasaki Disease Symposium, 2005

References

[1] *doctor/3259* (http://www.whonamedit.com/doctor.cfm/3259.html) at Who Named It?
[2] "Kawasaki Disease: Overview - eMedicine" (http://emedicine.medscape.com/article/352497-overview). . Retrieved 2009-01-04.
[3] Kawasaki T (March 1967). "[Acute febrile mucocutaneous syndrome with lymphoid involvement with specific desquamation of the fingers and toes in children]" (in Japanese). *Arerugi* **16** (3): 178–222. PMID 6062087 (http://www.ncbi.nlm.nih.gov/pubmed/6062087).
[4] Kawasaki T, Kosaki F, Okawa S, Shigematsu I, Yanagawa H (September 1974). "A new infantile acute febrile mucocutaneous lymph node syndrome (MLNS) prevailing in Japan". *Pediatrics* **54** (3): 271–6. PMID 4153258 (http://www.ncbi.nlm.nih.gov/pubmed/4153258).
[5] "Puzzling Peril for the Young" (http://www.time.com/time/magazine/article/0,9171,949010,00.html), *TIME Magazine*, U.S. Edition, **116** (8), August 25, 1980, , retrieved 2009-01-24

Heart

The **heart** is a muscular organ found in all vertebrates that is responsible for pumping blood throughout the blood vessels by repeated, rhythmic contractions. The term *cardiac* (as in cardiology) means "related to the heart" and comes from the Greek καρδιά, *kardia*, for "heart."

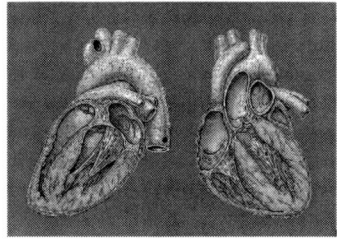

Heart

The vertebrate heart is composed of cardiac muscle, which is an involuntary striated muscle tissue found only within this organ. The average human heart, beating at 72 beats per minute, will beat approximately 2.5 billion times during an average 66 year lifespan. It weighs on average 250 g to 300 g in females and 300 g to 350 g in males.[1]

Early development

The mammalian heart is derived from embryonic mesoderm germ-layer cells that differentiate after gastrulation into mesothelium, endothelium, and myocardium. Mesothelial pericardium forms the outer lining of the heart. The inner lining of the heart, lymphatic and blood vessels, develop from endothelium. Myocardium develops into heart muscle.[2]

From splanchnopleuric mesoderm tissue, the cardiogenic plate develops cranially and laterally to the neural plate. In the cardiogenic plate, two separate angiogenic cell clusters form on either side of the embryo. Each cell cluster coalesces to form an endocardial tube continuous with a dorsal aorta and a vitteloumbilical vein. As embryonic tissue continues to fold, the two endocardial tubes are pushed into the thoracic cavity, begin to fuse together, and complete the fusing process at approximately 21 days.[3]

The human embryonic heart begins beating at around 21 days after conception, or five weeks after the last normal menstrual period (LMP). The first day of the LMP is normally used to date the start of the gestation (pregnancy). It is unknown how blood in the human embryo circulates for the first 21 days in the absence of a functioning heart. The human heart begins beating at a rate near the mother's, about 75-80 beats per minute (BPM).

The embryonic heart rate (EHR) then accelerates approximately 100 BPM during the first month of beating, peaking at 165-185 BPM during the early 7th week, (early 9th week after the LMP). This acceleration is approximately 3.3 BPM per day, or about 10 BPM every three days, which is an increase of 100 BPM in

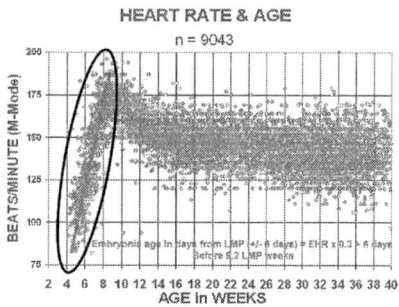

At 21 days after conception, the human heart begins beating at 70 to 80 beats per minute and accelerates linearly for the first month of beating.

the first month.[4] After 9.1 weeks after the LMP, it decelerates to about 152 BPM (+/-25 BPM) during the 15th week post LMP. After the 15th week, the deceleration slows to an average rate of about 145 (+/-25 BPM) BPM, at term. The regression formula, which describes this acceleration before the embryo reaches 25 mm in crown-rump length, or 9.2 LMP weeks, is: Age in days = EHR(0.3)+6. There is no difference in female and male heart rates before birth.[5]

Structure

The structure of the heart varies among the different branches of the animal kingdom. (See Circulatory system.) Cephalopods have two "gill hearts" and one "systemic heart". In vertebrates, the heart lies in the anterior part of the body cavity, dorsal to the gut. It is always surrounded by a pericardium, which is usually a distinct structure, but may be continuous with the peritoneum in jawless and cartilaginous fish. Hagfishes, uniquely among vertebrates, also possess a second heart-like structure in the tail.[6]

In humans

The heart is enclosed in a double-walled sac called the pericardium. The superficial part of this sac is called the fibrous pericardium. This sac protects the heart, anchors its surrounding structures, and prevents overfilling of the heart with blood. It is located anterior to the vertebral column and posterior to the sternum. The size of the heart is about the size of a fist and has a mass of between 250 grams and 350 grams. The heart is composed of three layers, all of which are rich with blood vessels. The superficial layer, called the visceral layer, the middle layer, called the myocardium, and the third layer which is called the endocardium. The heart has four chambers, two superior atria and two inferior ventricles. The atria are the receiving chambers and the ventricles are the discharging chambers. The pathway of blood through the heart consists of a pulmonary circuit and a systemic circuit. Blood flows through the heart in one direction, from the atrias to the ventricles, and out of the great arteries, or the aorta for example. This is done by four valves which are the tricuspid atrioventricular valve, the mitral atrioventricular valve, the aortic semilunar valve, and the pulmonary semilunar valve.[7]

In fish

Primitive fish have a four-chambered heart; however, the chambers are arranged sequentially so that this primitive heart is quite unlike the four-chambered hearts of mammals and birds. The first chamber is the sinus venosus, which collects de-oxygenated blood, from the body, through the hepatic and cardinal veins. From here, blood flows into the atrium and then to the powerful muscular ventricle where the main pumping action takes place. The fourth and final chamber is the conus arteriosus which contains several valves and sends blood to the *ventral aorta*. The ventral aorta delivers blood to the gills where it is oxygenated and flows, through the dorsal aorta, into the rest of the body. (In tetrapods, the ventral aorta has divided in two; one half forms the ascending aorta, while the other forms the pulmonary artery).[6]

In the adult fish, the four chambers are not arranged in a straight row but, instead, form an S-shape with the latter two chambers lying above the former two. This relatively simpler pattern is found in cartilaginous fish and in the more primitive ray-finned fish. In teleosts, the conus arteriosus is very small and can more accurately be described as part of the aorta rather than of the heart proper. The conus arteriosus is not present in any amniotes which presumably having been absorbed into the ventricles over the course of evolution. Similarly, while the sinus venosus is present as a vestigial structure in some reptiles and birds, it is otherwise absorbed into the right atrium and is no longer distinguishable.[6]

In double circulatory systems

In amphibians and most reptiles, a double circulatory system is used but the heart is not completely separated into two pumps. The development of the double system is necessitated by the presence of lungs which deliver oxygenated blood directly to the heart.

In living amphibians, the atrium is divided into two separate chambers by the presence of a muscular septum even though there is only a single ventricle. The sinus venosus, which remains large in amphibians but connects only to the right atrium, receives blood from the vena cavae, with the pulmonary vein by-passing it entirely to enter the left atrium.

In the heart of lungfish, the septum extends part-way into the ventricle. This allows for some degree of separation between the de-oxygenated bloodstream destined for the lungs and the oxygenated stream that is delivered to the rest of the body. The absence of such a division in living amphibian species may be at least partly due to the amount of respiration that occurs through the skin in such species; thus, the blood returned to the heart through the vena cavae is, in fact, already partially oxygenated. As a result, there may be less need for a finer division between the two bloodstreams than in lungfish or other tetrapods. Nonetheless, in at least some species of amphibian, the spongy nature of the ventricle seems to maintain more of a separation between the bloodstreams than appears the case at first glance. Furthermore, the conus arteriosus has lost its original valves and contains a spiral valve, instead, that divides it into two parallel parts, thus helping to keep the two bloodstreams separate.[6]

The heart of most reptiles (except for crocodilians; *see below*) has a similar structure to that of lungfish but, here, the septum is generally much larger. This divides the ventricle into two halves but, because the septum does not reach the whole length of the heart, there is a considerable gap near the openings to the pulmonary artery and the aorta. In practice, however, in the majority of reptilian species, there appears to be little, if any, mixing between the bloodstreams that the aorta receives, essentially, only oxygenated blood.[6]

The fully-divided heart

Archosaurs, (crocodilians, birds), and mammals show complete separation of the heart into two pumps for a total of four heart chambers; it is thought that the four-chambered heart of archosaurs evolved independently from that of mammals. In crocodilians, there is a small opening, the foramen of Panizza, at the base of the arterial trunks and there is some degree of mixing between the blood in each side of the heart; thus, only in birds and mammals are the two streams of blood - those to the pulmonary and systemic circulations - kept entirely separate by a physical barrier.[6]

In the human body, the heart is usually situated in the middle of the thorax with the largest part of the heart slightly offset to the left, although sometimes it is on the right (see dextrocardia), underneath the sternum. The heart is usually felt to be on the left side because the left heart (left ventricle) is stronger (it pumps to all body parts). The left lung is smaller than the right lung because the heart occupies more of the left hemithorax. The heart is fed by the coronary circulation and is enclosed by a sac known as the pericardium; it is also surrounded by the lungs. The pericardium comprises two parts: the fibrous pericardium, made of dense fibrous connective tissue, and a double membrane structure (parietal and visceral pericardium) containing a serous fluid to reduce friction during heart contractions. The heart is located in the mediastinum, which is the central sub-division of the thoracic cavity. The mediastinum also contains other structures, such as the esophagus and trachea, and is flanked on either side by the right and left pulmonary cavities; these cavities house the lungs.[9]

The *apex* is the blunt point situated in an inferior (pointing down and left) direction. A stethoscope can be placed directly over the apex so that the beats can be counted. It is located posterior to the 5th intercostal space just medial of the left mid-clavicular line. In normal adults, the mass of the heart is 250-350 g (9-12 oz), or about twice the size of a clenched fist (it is about the size of a clenched fist in children), but an extremely diseased heart can be up to 1000 g (2 lb) in mass due to hypertrophy. It consists of four chambers, the two upper atria and the two lower ventricles.

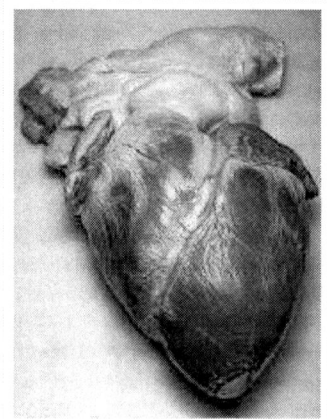
Human heart removed from a 64-year-old male.

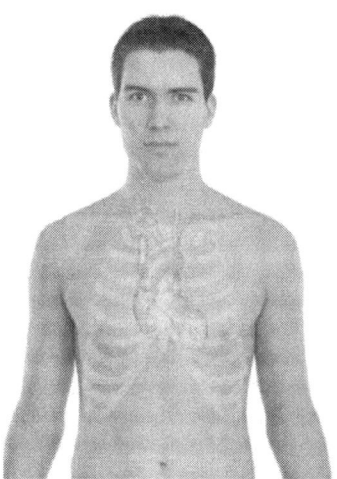
Surface anatomy of the human heart. The heart is demarcated by:
-A point 9 cm to the left of the midsternal line (apex of the heart)
-The seventh right sternocostal articulation
-The upper border of the third right costal cartilage 1 cm from the right sternal line
-The lower border of the second left costal cartilage 2.5 cm from the left lateral sternal line.[8]

Functioning

In mammals, the function of the right side of the heart (see right heart) is to collect de-oxygenated blood, in the right atrium, from the body (via superior and inferior vena cavae) and pump it, via the right ventricle, into the lungs (pulmonary circulation) so that carbon dioxide can be dropped off and oxygen picked up (gas exchange). This happens through the passive process of diffusion. The left side (see left heart) collects oxygenated blood from the lungs into the left atrium. From the left atrium the blood moves to the left ventricle which pumps it out to the body (via the aorta). On both sides, the lower ventricles are thicker and stronger than the upper atria. The muscle wall surrounding the left ventricle is thicker than the wall surrounding the right ventricle due to the higher force needed to pump the blood through the systemic circulation.

Starting in the right atrium, the blood flows through the tricuspid valve to the right ventricle. Here, it is pumped out the pulmonary semilunar valve and travels through the pulmonary artery to the lungs. From there, blood flows back through the pulmonary vein to the left atrium. It then travels through the mitral valve to the left ventricle, from where it is pumped through the aortic semilunar valve to the aorta. The aorta forks and the blood is divided between major arteries which supply the upper and lower body. The blood travels in the arteries to the smaller arterioles and then, finally, to the tiny capillaries which feed each cell. The (relatively) deoxygenated blood then travels to the venules, which coalesce into veins, then to the inferior and superior venae cavae and finally back to the right atrium where the process began.

The heart is effectively a syncytium, a meshwork of cardiac muscle cells interconnected by contiguous cytoplasmic bridges. This relates to electrical stimulation of one cell spreading to neighboring cells.

Some cardiac cells are self-excitable, contracting without any signal from the nervous system, even if removed from the heart and placed in culture. Each of these cells have their own intrinsic contraction rhythm. A region of the human heart called the **sinoatrial node**, or pacemaker, sets the rate and timing at which all cardiac muscle cells contract. The SA node generates electrical impulses, much like those produced by nerve cells. Because cardiac muscle cells are electrically coupled by inter-calated disks between adjacent cells, impulses from the SA node spread rapidly through the walls of the artria, causing both artria to contract in unison. The impulses also pass to another region of specialized cardiac muscle tissue, a relay point called the **atrioventricular node**, located in the wall between the right artrium and the right ventricle. Here, the impulses are delayed for about 0.1s before spreading to the walls of the ventricle. The delay ensures that the artria empty completely before the ventricles contract. Specialized muscle fibers called Purkinje fibers then conduct the signals to the apex of the heart along and throughout the ventricular walls. The Purkinje fibres form conducting pathways called bundle branches. This entire cycle, a single heart beat, lasts about 0.8 seconds. The impulses generated during the heart cycle produce electrical currents, which are conducted through body fluids to the skin, where they can be detected by electrodes and recorded as an electrocardiogram (ECG or EKG).[10]

The SA node is found in all amniotes but not in more primitive vertebrates. In these animals, the muscles of the heart are relatively continuous and the sinus venosus coordinates the beat which passes in a wave through the remaining chambers. Indeed, since the sinus venosus is incorporated into the right atrium in amniotes, it is likely homologous with the SA node. In teleosts, with their vestigial sinus venosus, the main centre of coordination is, instead, in the atrium. The rate of heartbeat varies enormously between different species, ranging from around 20 beats per minute in codfish to around 600 in hummingbirds.[6]

Cardiac arrest is the sudden cessation of normal heart rhythm which can include a number of pathologies such as tachycardia, an extremely rapid heart beat which prevents the heart from effectively pumping blood, fibrillation, which is an irregular and ineffective heart rhythm, and asystole, which is the cessation of heart rhythm entirely.

Cardiac tamponade is a condition in which the fibrous sac surrounding the heart fills with excess fluid or blood, suppressing the heart's ability to beat properly. Tamponade is treated by pericardiocentesis, the gentle insertion of the needle of a syringe into the pericardial sac (avoiding the heart itself) on an angle, usually from just below the sternum, and gently withdrawing the tamponading fluids.

History of discoveries

The valves of the heart were discovered by a physician of the Hippocratean school around the 4th century BC. However, their function was not properly understood then. Because blood pools in the veins after death, arteries look empty. Ancient anatomists assumed they were filled with air and that they were for transport of air.

Philosophers distinguished veins from arteries but thought that the pulse was a property of arteries themselves. Erasistratos observed the arteries that were cut during life bleed. He described the fact to the phenomenon that air escaping from an artery is replaced with blood which entered by very small vessels between veins and arteries. Thus he apparently postulated capillaries but with reversed flow of blood.

The 2nd century AD, Greek physician Galenos (Galen) knew that blood vessels carried blood and identified venous (dark red) and arterial (brighter and thinner) blood, each with distinct and separate functions. Growth and energy were derived from venous blood created in the liver from chyle, while arterial blood gave vitality by containing pneuma (air) and originated in the heart. Blood flowed from both creating organs to all parts of the body where it was consumed and there was no return of blood to the heart or liver. The heart did not pump blood around, the heart's motion sucked blood in during diastole and the blood moved by the pulsation of the arteries themselves.

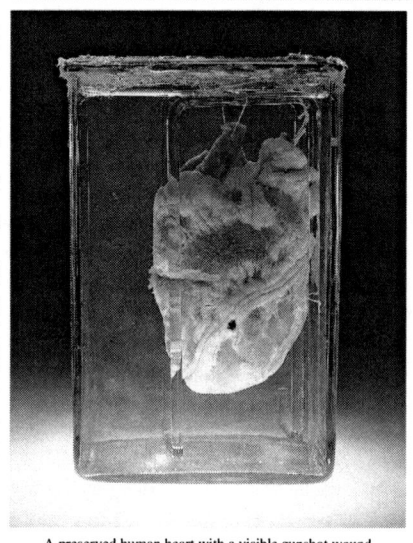

A preserved human heart with a visible gunshot wound

Galen believed that the arterial blood was created by venous blood passing from the left ventricle to the right through 'pores' in the inter ventricular septum while air passed from the lungs via the pulmonary artery to the left side of the heart. As the arterial blood was created, 'sooty' vapors were created and passed to the lungs, also via the pulmonary artery, to be exhaled.

The first major scientific understanding of the heart was put forth by the medieval Arab polymath Ibn Al-Nafis, regarded as the father of circulatory physiology.[11] He was the first physician to correctly describe pulmonary circulation,[12] the capillary[13] and coronary circulations.[14] Prior to this, Galen's theory was widely accepted, and improved upon by Avicenna. Al-Nafis rejected the Galen-Avicenna theory and corrected many wrong ideas that were put forth by it, and also adding his new found observations of pulse and circulation to the new theory. His major observations include (as surmised by Dr. Paul Ghalioungui):[13]

1. "Denying the existence of any pores through the interventricular septum."
2. "The flow of blood from the right ventricle to the lungs where its lighter parts filter into the pulmonary vein to mix with air."
3. "The notion that blood, or spirit from the mixture of blood and air, passes from the lung to the left ventricle, and not in the opposite direction."
4. "The assertion that there are only two ventricles, not three as stated by Avicenna."
5. "The statement that the ventricle takes its nourishment from blood flowing in the vessels that run in its substance (i.e. the coronary vessels) and not, as Avicenna maintained, from blood deposited in the right ventricle."
6. "A premonition of the capillary circulation in his assertion that the pulmonary vein receives what comes out of the pulmonary artery, this being the reason for the existence of perceptible passages between the two."

Ibn Al-Nafis also corrected Galen-Avicenna assertion that heart has a bone structure through his own observations and wrote the following criticism on it:[15]

> "This is not true. There are absolutely no bones beneath the heart as it is positioned right in the middle of the chest cavity where there are no bones at all. Bones are only found at the chest periphery not where the heart is positioned."

For more recent technological developments, see Cardiac surgery.

Healthy heart

Obesity, high blood pressure, and high cholesterol can increase the risk of developing heart disease. However, fully half the amount of heart attacks occur in people with normal cholesterol levels. Heart disease is a major cause of death (and the number one cause of death in the Western World).

Of course one must also consider other factors such as lifestyle, for instance the amount of exercise one undertakes and their diet, as well as their overall health (mental and social as well as physical).[16] [17] [18] [19]

See also

- Cardiac cycle
- Heart disease
- Human heart
- Electrocardiogram
- Electrical conduction system of the heart
- Physiology
- Trauma triad of death

External links

- Heart contraction and blood flow (animation) [20]
- Heart Disease [21]
- eMedicine: Surgical anatomy of the heart [22]
- Interactive 3D heart [23] This realistic heart can be rotated, and all its components can be studied from any angle.
- Heart Information [24]

References

[1] Kumar, Abbas, Fausto: *Robbins and Cotran Pathologic Basis of Disease*, 7th Ed. p. 556
[2] Animal Tissues (http://users.rcn.com/jkimball.ma.ultranet/BiologyPages/A/AnimalTissues.html)
[3] Main Frame Heart Development> (http://www.meddean.luc.edu/lumen/MedEd/GrossAnatomy/thorax0/heartdev/main_fra.html)
[4] OBGYN.net "Embryonic Heart Rates Compared in Assisted and Non-Assisted Pregnancies" (http://www.obgyn.net/us/us.asp?page=/us/cotm/0001/ehr2000)
[5] Terry J. DuBose Sex, Heart Rate and Age (http://www.obgyn.net/english/pubs/features/dubose/ehr-age.htm)
[6] Romer, Alfred Sherwood; Parsons, Thomas S. (1977). *The Vertebrate Body*. Philadelphia, PA: Holt-Saunders International. pp. 437–442. ISBN 0-03-910284-X.
[7] Marieb, Elaine Nicpon. Human Anatomy & Physiology. 6th ed. Upper Saddle River: Pearson Education, 2003. Print
[8] Gray's Anatomy of the Human Body - 6. Surface Markings of the Thorax (http://www.bartleby.com/107/284.html)
[9] Maton, Anthea; Jean Hopkins, Charles William McLaughlin, Susan Johnson, Maryanna Quon Warner, David LaHart, Jill D. Wright (1993). *Human Biology and Health*. Englewood Cliffs, New Jersey: Prentice Hall. ISBN 0-13-981176-1. OCLC 32308337 (http://worldcat.org/oclc/32308337).
[10] Campbell, Reece-Biology, 7th Ed. p.873,874
[11] Chairman's Reflections (2004), "Traditional Medicine Among Gulf Arabs, Part II: Blood-letting", Heart Views 5 (2): 74-85 [80]
[12] S. A. Al-Dabbagh (1978). "Ibn Al-Nafis and the pulmonary circulation", The Lancet 1: 1148

[13] (http://www.islamset.com/isc/nafis/drpaul.html) Dr. Paul Ghalioungui (1982), "The West denies Ibn Al Nafis's contribution to the discovery of the circulation", *Symposium on Ibn al-Nafis*, Second International Conference on Islamic Medicine: Islamic Medical Organization, Kuwait (cf.) The West denies Ibn Al Nafis's contribution to the discovery of the circulation
[14] Husain F. Nagamia (2003), "Ibn al-Nafis: A Biographical Sketch of the Discoverer of Pulmonary and Coronary Circulation", Journal of the International Society for the History of Islamic Medicine 1: 22–28.
[15] Dr. Sulaiman Oataya (1982), "Ibn ul Nafis has dissected the human body", Symposium on Ibn al-Nafis, Second International Conference on Islamic Medicine: Islamic Medical Organization, Kuwait (cf. Ibn ul-Nafis has Dissected the Human Body, Encyclopedia of Islamic World).
[16] "Eating for a healthy heart" (http://www.medicineweb.com/nutrition-/eating-for-a-healthy-heart). MedicineWeb. . Retrieved 2009-03-31.
[17] Division of Vital Statistics; Arialdi M. Miniño, M.P.H., Melonie P. Heron, Ph.D., Sherry L. Murphy, B.S., Kenneth D. Kochanek, M.A. (2007-08-21). "Deaths: Final data for 2004" (http://www.cdc.gov/nchs/data/nvsr/nvsr55/nvsr55_19.pdf) (PDF). *National Vital Statistics Reports* (United States: Center for Disease Control) **55** (19): 7. . Retrieved 2007-12-30.
[18] White House News. "American Heart Month, 2007" (http://georgewbush-whitehouse.archives.gov/news/releases/2007/02/20070201-2.html). . Retrieved 2007-07-16.
[19] National Statistics Press Release (http://www.statistics.gov.uk/pdfdir/hsq0506.pdf) 25 May 2006
[20] http://www.nhlbi.nih.gov/health/dci/Diseases/hhw/hhw_pumping.html
[21] http://www.heart.org.in/
[22] http://www.emedicine.com/ped/topic2902.htm
[23] http://thevirtualheart.org/anatomyindex.html
[24] http://www.pharmacyproductinfo.com/Heart.html

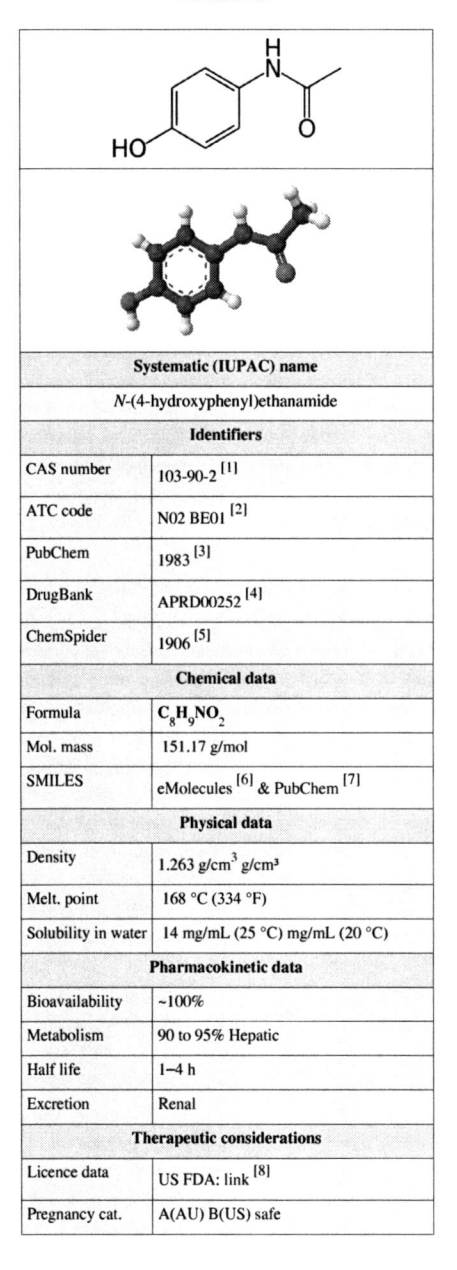

Paracetamol

Paracetamol

Systematic (IUPAC) name	
N-(4-hydroxyphenyl)ethanamide	
Identifiers	
CAS number	103-90-2 [1]
ATC code	N02 BE01 [2]
PubChem	1983 [3]
DrugBank	APRD00252 [4]
ChemSpider	1906 [5]
Chemical data	
Formula	$C_8H_9NO_2$
Mol. mass	151.17 g/mol
SMILES	eMolecules [6] & PubChem [7]
Physical data	
Density	1.263 g/cm³ g/cm³
Melt. point	168 °C (334 °F)
Solubility in water	14 mg/mL (25 °C) mg/mL (20 °C)
Pharmacokinetic data	
Bioavailability	~100%
Metabolism	90 to 95% Hepatic
Half life	1–4 h
Excretion	Renal
Therapeutic considerations	
Licence data	US FDA: link [8]
Pregnancy cat.	A(AU) B(US) safe

Legal status	Unscheduled (AU) GSL (UK) OTC (US)
Routes	Oral, rectal, intravenous

✓ (what is this?) (verify) [9]

Paracetamol (INN) (pronounced /ˌpærəˈsiːtəmɒl/, ˌpærəˈsɛtəmɒl/) or **acetaminophen** (English pronunciation: /əˌsiːtəˈmɪnəfɪn/ (◄» listen)) (USAN) is a widely used over-the-counter analgesic (pain reliever) and antipyretic (fever reducer). It is commonly used for the relief of fever, headaches, and other minor aches and pains, and is a major ingredient in numerous cold and flu remedies. In combination with non-steroidal anti-inflammatory drugs (NSAIDs) and opioid analgesics, paracetamol is used also in the management of more severe pain (such as postoperative pain).[10]

While generally safe for human use at recommended doses (1000 mg per single dose and up to 4000 mg per day for adults, up to 2000 mg per day if drinking alcohol[11]), acute overdoses of paracetamol can cause potentially fatal liver damage and, in rare individuals, a normal dose can do the same; the risk is heightened by alcohol consumption. Paracetamol toxicity is the foremost cause of acute liver failure in the Western world, and accounts for most drug overdoses in the United States, the United Kingdom, Australia and New Zealand.[12] [13] [14] [15]

Paracetamol is derived from coal tar, and is part of the class of drugs known as "aniline analgesics"; it is the only such drug still in use today.[16] It is the active metabolite of phenacetin, once popular as an analgesic and antipyretic in its own right, but unlike phenacetin and its combinations, paracetamol is not considered to be carcinogenic at therapeutic doses.[17] The words *acetaminophen* (used in the United States, Canada, Hong Kong, Iran[18] , Colombia and other Latin American countries) and *paracetamol* (used elsewhere) both come from chemical names for the compound: *para*-**acet**yl**amino**phen**ol** and *para*-**acet**yl**am**ino**phen**ol**. In some contexts, it is simply abbreviated as **APAP**, for *N*-acetyl-para-aminophenol.

History

Acetanilide was the first aniline derivative serendipitously found to possess analgesic as well as antipyretic properties, and was quickly introduced into medical practice under the name of Antifebrin by A. Cahn and P. Hepp in 1886.[19] But its unacceptable toxic effects, the most alarming being cyanosis due to methemoglobinemia, prompted the search for less toxic aniline derivatives.[16] Harmon Northrop Morse had already synthesized paracetamol at Johns Hopkins University via the reduction of *p*-nitrophenol with tin in glacial acetic acid in 1877,[20] [21] but it wasn't until 1887 that clinical pharmacologist Joseph von Mering tried paracetamol on patients.[16] In 1893, von Mering published a paper reporting on the clinical results of paracetamol with phenacetin, another aniline derivative.[22] Von Mering claimed that, unlike phenacetin, paracetamol had a slight tendency to produce methemoglobinemia. Paracetamol was then quickly discarded in favor of phenacetin. The sales of phenacetin established Bayer as a leading pharmaceutical company.[23] Overshadowed in part by aspirin, introduced into medicine by Heinrich Dreser in 1899, phenacetin was popular for many decades, particularly in widely advertised over-the-counter "headache mixtures," usually containing phenacetin, an aminopyrine derivative or aspirin, caffeine, and sometimes a barbiturate.[16]

Von Mering's claims remained essentially unchallenged for half a century, until two teams of researchers from the United States analyzed the metabolism of acetanilide and paracetamol.[23] In 1947 David Lester and Leon Greenberg found strong evidence that paracetamol was a major metabolite of acetanilide in human blood, and in a subsequent study they reported that large doses of paracetamol given to albino rats did not cause methemoglobinemia.[24] In three papers published in the September 1948 issue of the *Journal of Pharmacology and Experimental Therapeutics*, Bernard Brodie, Julius Axelrod and Frederick Flinn confirmed using more specific methods that paracetamol was the major metabolite of acetanilide in human blood, and established it was just as efficacious an analgesic as its precursor.[25] [26] [27] They also suggested that methemoglobinemia is produced in humans mainly by another metabolite, phenylhydroxylamine. A followup paper by Brodie and Axelrod in 1949 established that phenacetin was also metabolized to paracetamol.[28] This led to a "rediscovery" of paracetamol.[16] It has been suggested that contamination of paracetamol with 4-aminophenol, the substance from which it was synthesized by von Mering, may be the cause for his spurious findings.[23]

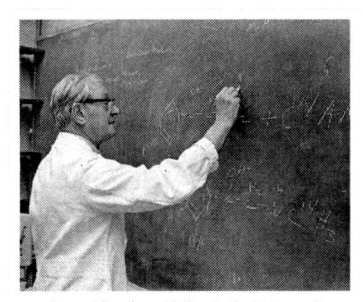

Paracetamol was first marketed in the United States in 1953 by Sterling-Winthrop Co., which promoted it as preferable to aspirin since it was safe to take for children and people with ulcers.[23] The best known brand today for paracetamol in the United States, Tylenol, was established in 1955 when McNeil Laboratories started selling paracetamol as a pain and fever reliever for children, under the brand name Tylenol Children's Elixir—the word "tylenol" was a contraction of *para*-acetylaminophenol.[29] In 1956, 500 mg tablets of paracetamol went on sale in the United Kingdom under the trade name Panadol, produced by Frederick Stearns & Co, a subsidiary of Sterling Drug Inc. Panadol was originally available only by prescription, for the relief of pain and fever, and was advertised as being "gentle to the stomach," since other analgesic agents of the time contained aspirin, a known stomach irritant. In 1963, paracetamol was added to the *British Pharmacopoeia*, and has gained popularity since then as an analgesic agent with few side-effects and little interaction with other pharmaceutical agents.[21] Concerns about paracetamol's safety delayed its widespread acceptance until the 1970s, but in the 1980s paracetamol sales exceeded those of aspirin in many countries, including the United Kingdom. This was accompanied by the commercial demise of phenacetin, blamed as the cause of analgesic nephropathy and hematological toxicity.[16]

Bernard Brodie and Julius Axelrod *(pictured)* demonstrated that acetanilide and phenacetin are both metabolized to paracetamol, which is a better tolerated analgesic.

The U.S. patent on paracetamol has long expired, and generic versions of the drug are widely available under the Drug Price Competition and Patent Term Restoration Act of 1984, although certain Tylenol preparations were protected until 2007. U.S. patent 6,126,967 filed September 3, 1998 was granted for "Extended release acetaminophen particles".[30]

Structure and reactivity

Paracetamol consists of a benzene ring core, substituted by one hydroxyl group and the nitrogen atom of an amide group in the *para* (1,4) pattern.[31] The amide group is acetamide (ethanamide). It is an extensively conjugated system, as the lone pair on the hydroxyl oxygen, the benzene pi cloud, the nitrogen lone pair, the p orbital on the carbonyl carbon, and the lone pair on the carbonyl oxygen are all conjugated. The presence of two activating groups also make the benzene ring highly reactive toward electrophilic aromatic substitution. As the substituents are ortho,para-directing and para with respect to each other, all positions on the ring are more or less equally activated.

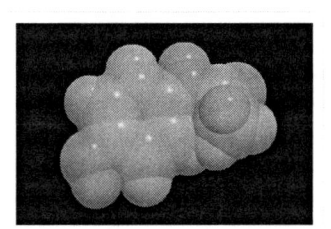

Polar surface area of the paracetamol molecule

The conjugation also greatly reduces the basicity of the oxygens and the nitrogen, while making the hydroxyl acidic through delocalisation of charge developed on the phenoxide anion.

Synthesis

Compared with many other drugs, paracetamol is much easier to synthesize, because it lacks stereocenters. As a result, there is no need to design a stereo-selective synthesis.

Industrial preparation of paracetamol usually proceeds from nitrobenzene.[32] A one-step reductive acetamidation reaction can be mediated by thioacetate.[33]

Paracetamol may be easily prepared in the laboratory by nitrating phenol with sodium nitrate, separating the desired *p*-nitrophenol from the *ortho*- byproduct, and reducing the nitro group with sodium borohydride. The resultant *p*-aminophenol is then acetylated with acetic anhydride.[34] In this reaction, phenol is strongly activating, thus the reaction only requires mild conditions (c.f. the nitration of benzene):

Reactions

p-Aminophenol may be obtained by the amide hydrolysis of paracetamol. *p*-Aminophenol prepared this way, and related to the commercially available Metol, has been used as a developer in photography by hobbyists.[35]

Available forms

Paracetamol is available in a tablet, capsule, liquid suspension, suppository, intravenous, and intramuscular form. The common adult dose is 500 mg to 1000 mg. The recommended maximum daily dose, for adults, is 4000 mg. In recommended doses, paracetamol generally is safe for children and infants, as well as for adults.[36]

Panadol, which is marketed in Africa, Asia, Central America, and Australasia, is the most widely available brand, sold in over 80 countries. In North America, paracetamol is sold in generic form (usually labeled as acetaminophen) or under a number of trade names, for instance, **Tylenol** (McNeil-PPC, Inc.),**Tydenol** (Edruc

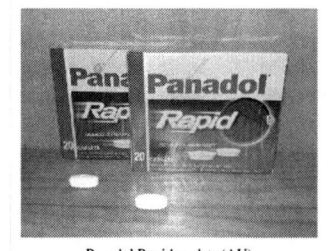

Panadol Rapid caplets (AU)

Limited,Bangladesh) **Anacin-3**, **Tempra**, and **Datril**,. While there is brand named paracetamol available in the UK (e.g. Panadol), unbranded or generic paracetamol is more commonly sold. **Acamol**, a brand name for paracetamol produced by Teva Pharmaceutical Industries in Israel, is one of the most popular drugs in that country. In Europe, the most common brands of paracetamol are **Efferalgan** and **Doliprane**. In India, the most common brand of paracetamol is **Crocin** manufactured by Glaxo SmithKline Asia. In Bangladesh the most popular brand is **Napa** manufactured by Beximco Pharma.

In some formulations, paracetamol is combined with the opioid codeine, sometimes referred to as co-codamol (BAN). In the United States and Canada, this is marketed under the name of Tylenol #1/2/3/4, which contain 8–10 mg, 15 mg, 30 mg, and 60 mg of codeine, respectively. In the U.S., this combination is available only by prescription, while the lowest-strength preparation is over-the-counter in Canada, and, in other countries, other strengths may be available over the counter. There are generic forms of these combinations as well. In the UK and in many other countries, this combination is marketed under the names of Tylex CD and Panadeine. Other names include Captin, Disprol, Dymadon, Fensum, Hedex, Mexalen, Nofedol, Paralen, Pediapirin, Perfalgan, and Solpadeine. Paracetamol is also combined with other opioids such as dihydrocodeine, referred to as co-dydramol (BAN), oxycodone or hydrocodone, marketed in the U.S. as Percocet and Vicodin, respectively. Another very commonly used analgesic combination includes paracetamol in combination with propoxyphene napsylate, sold under the brand name Darvocet. A combination of paracetamol, codeine, and the calmative doxylamine succinate is marketed as Syndol or Mersyndol.

Paracetamol is commonly used in multi-ingredient preparations for migraine headache, typically including butalbital and paracetamol with or without caffeine, and sometimes containing codeine.

Brand Names[37]

Aceta, Actimin, Anacin-3, Apacet, Aspirin Free Anacin, Atasol, Banesin, Ben-uron, Crocin, Dapa, Dolo, Datril Extra-Strength, DayQuil, Depon & Depon Maximum, Feverall, Few Drops, Fibi, Fibi plus, Genapap, Genebs, Lekadol, LemSip, Liquiprin, Lupocet, Neopap, Ny-Quil, Oraphen-PD, Panado, Panadol, Paracet, Paralen, Phenaphen, Plicet, Redutemp, Snaplets-FR, Suppap, Tamen, Tapanol, Tempra, Tylenol, Valorin, Xcel.

Mechanism of action

Paracetamol is usually classified along with nonsteroidal antiinflammatory drugs (NSAID), but is not considered one, rather is part of the class of drugs known as aniline analgesics. Like all drugs of this class, its main mechanism of action is the inhibition of cyclooxygenase (COX), an enzyme responsible for the production of prostaglandins, which are important mediators of inflammation, pain and fever. Therefore, all NSAIDs are said to possess anti-inflammatory, analgesic (anti-pain), and antipyretic (anti-fever) properties. The specific actions of each NSAID drug depends upon their pharmacological properties, distribution and metabolism.

While paracetamol has analgesic and antipyretic properties comparable to those of aspirin, it fails to exert significant anti-inflammatory action due to paracetamol's susceptibility to the high level of peroxides present in inflammatory lesions.

However, the mechanism by which paracetamol reduces fever and pain is still debated[38] largely because paracetamol reduces the production of prostaglandins (pro-inflammatory chemicals). Aspirin also inhibits the production of prostaglandins, but, unlike aspirin, paracetamol has little anti-inflammatory action. Likewise, whereas aspirin inhibits the production of the pro-clotting chemicals thromboxanes, paracetamol does not. Aspirin is known to inhibit the cyclooxygenase (COX) family of enzymes, and, because of paracetamol's partial similarity of aspirin's action, much research has focused on whether paracetamol also inhibits COX. It is now clear that paracetamol acts via at least two pathways.[16] [39] [40] [41]

AM404—a metabolite of paracetamol

The COX family of enzymes are responsible for the metabolism of arachidonic acid to prostaglandin H$_2$, an unstable molecule, which is, in turn, converted to numerous other pro-inflammatory compounds. Classical anti-inflammatories, such as the NSAIDs, block this step. Only when appropriately oxidized is the COX enzyme highly active.[42] [43] Paracetamol reduces the oxidized form of the COX enzyme, preventing it from forming pro-inflammatory chemicals.[40] [44]. Thus reducing the amount of *Prostaglandin E2* in the CNS and thus lowering the hypothalamic set point in the thermoregulatory centre. Inhibition of another enzyme **COX3** is specifically implicated in the case of paracetamol. COX3 is not seen outside the CNS Article text.[45] Paracetamol also modulates the endogenous cannabinoid system.[46] Paracetamol is metabolized to AM404, a compound with several actions; most important, it inhibits the uptake of the endogenous cannabinoid/vanilloid anandamide by neurons. Anandamide uptake would result in the activation of the main pain receptor (nociceptor) of the body, the TRPV1 (older name: vanilloid receptor). Furthermore, AM404 inhibits sodium channels, as do the anesthetics lidocaine and procaine.[47] Either of these actions by themselves has been shown to reduce pain, and are a possible mechanism for paracetamol, though it has been demonstrated that, after blocking cannabinoid receptors and hence making any action of cannabinoid reuptake irrelevant, paracetamol loses analgesic effect, suggesting its pain-relieving action is mediated by the endogenous cannabinoid system.[48]

Anandamide—an endogenous cannabinoid

One theory holds that paracetamol works by inhibiting the COX-3 isoform of the COX family of enzymes. This enzyme, when expressed in dogs, shares a strong similarity to the other COX enzymes, produces pro-inflammatory chemicals, and is selectively inhibited by paracetamol.[49] However, some research has suggested that in humans and mice, the COX-3 enzyme is without inflammatory action.[39] Another possibility is that paracetamol blocks cyclooxygenase (as in aspirin), but that in an inflammatory environment, where the concentration of peroxides is high, the oxidation state of paracetamol is high which prevents its actions. This would mean that paracetamol has no direct effect at the site of inflammation but instead acts in the CNS to reduce temperature etc where the environment is not oxidative.[49] The exact mechanism by which paracetamol is believed to affect COX-3 is disputed.

Metabolism

Paracetamol is metabolised primarily in the liver, into non-toxic products. Three metabolic pathways are notable:

- Glucuronidation is believed to account for 40% to two-thirds of the metabolism of paracetamol.[50]
- Sulfation (sulfate conjugation) may account for 20–40%.[50]
- N-hydroxylation and rearrangement, then GSH conjugation, accounts for less than 15%. The hepatic cytochrome P450 enzyme system metabolizes paracetamol, forming a minor yet significant alkylating metabolite known as NAPQI (*N*-acetyl-*p*-benzo-quinone imine).[51] NAPQI is then irreversibly conjugated with the sulfhydryl groups of glutathione.[51]

All three pathways yield final products that are inactive, non-toxic, and eventually excreted by the kidneys. In the third pathway, however, the intermediate product NAPQI is toxic. NAPQI is primarily responsible for the toxic effects of paracetamol; this constitutes an excellent example of toxication.

Main pathways of paracetamol metabolism (click to enlarge). Pathways shown in blue and purple lead to non-toxic metabolites; the pathway in red leads to toxic NAPQI.

Production of NAPQI is due primarily to two isoenzymes of cytochrome P450: CYP2E1 and CYP1A2. The P450 gene is highly polymorphic, however, and individual differences in paracetamol toxicity are believed to be due to a third isoenzyme, CYP2D6. Genetic polymorphisms in CYP2D6 may contribute to significantly different rates of production of NAPQI. Furthermore, individuals can be classified as "extensive", "ultrarapid", and "poor" metabolizers (producers of NAPQI), depending on their levels of CYP2D6 expression. Although CYP2D6 metabolises paracetamol into NAPQI to a lesser extent than other P450 enzymes, its activity may contribute to paracetamol toxicity in extensive and ultrarapid metabolisers, and when paracetamol is taken at very large doses.[52] At usual doses, NAPQI is quickly detoxified by conjugation.[51] Following overdose, and possibly also in extensive and ultrarapid metabolizers, this detoxification pathway becomes saturated and consequently NAPQI accumulates.

Indications

The WHO recommends that paracetamol be given to children with fever higher than 38.5°C (101.3°F).[53]

Paracetamol is a suitable substitute for aspirin, especially in patients where excessive gastric acid secretion or prolongation of bleeding time may be a concern. While paracetamol has analgesic and antipyretic properties comparable to those of aspirin, its anti-inflammatory effects are weak. Because paracetamol is well tolerated, available without a prescription, and lacks the gastric side effects of aspirin, it has in recent years increasingly become a common household drug.

Efficacy and side effects

Paracetamol, unlike other common analgesics such as aspirin and ibuprofen, has relatively little anti-inflammatory activity, so it is *not* considered to be a non-steroidal anti-inflammatory drug (NSAID).

Efficacy

Regarding comparative efficacy, studies show conflicting results when compared to NSAIDs. A randomized controlled trial of chronic pain from osteoarthritis in adults found similar benefit from paracetamol and ibuprofen.[54] [55] However, a randomized controlled trial of acute musculoskeletal pain in children found that the standard OTC dose of ibuprofen gives greater relief of pain than the standard dose of paracetamol.[56]

Adverse effects

In recommended doses, paracetamol does not irritate the lining of the stomach, affect blood coagulation as much as NSAIDs, or affect function of the kidneys. However, some studies have shown that high dose-usage (greater than 2,000 mg per day) does increase the risk of upper gastrointestinal complications such as stomach bleeding.[57] The researchers found that heavy use of aspirin or paracetamol - defined as 300 grams a year (1 g per day on average) - was linked to a condition known as small, indented and calcified kidneys (SICK).[58] Paracetamol is safe in pregnancy, and does not affect the closure of the fetal ductus arteriosus as NSAIDs can.[59] Unlike aspirin, it is safe in children, as paracetamol is not associated with a risk of Reye's syndrome in children with viral illnesses.[60]

Like NSAIDs and unlike opioid analgesics, paracetamol has not been found to cause euphoria or alter mood in any way. In 2008, the largest study to date on the long term side effects of paracetamol in children was published in The Lancet. Conducted on over 200,000 children in 31 countries, the study found that the use of paracetamol for fever in the first year of life was associated with an increase in the incidence of asthmatic symptoms at 6–7 years, and that paracetamol use, both in the first year of life and in children aged 6–7 years, was associated with an increased incidence of rhinoconjunctivitis and eczema.[61] The authors acknowledged that their "findings might have been due to confounding by indication", i.e. that the association may not be causal but rather due to the disease being treated with paracetamol, and emphasized that further research was needed. Furthermore a number of editorials, comments, correspondence and their replies have been published in The Lancet concerning the methodology and conclusions of this study.[62] [63] [64] [65] [66] [67] [68] The UK regulatory body the Medicines and Healthcare products Regulatory Agency, also reviewed this research and published a number of concerns over data interpretation, and offer the following advice for healthcare professionals, parents, and carers: "The results of this new study do not necessitate any change to the current guidance for use in children. Paracetamol remains a safe and appropriate choice of analgesic in children. There is insufficient evidence from this research to change guidance regarding the use of antipyretics in children."[69]

Toxicity

Excessive use of paracetamol can damage multiple organs, especially the liver and kidney. In both organs, toxicity from paracetamol is not from the drug itself but from one of its metabolites, *N*-acetyl-*p*-benzoquinoneimine (NAPQI). In the liver, the cytochrome P450 enzymes CYP2E1 and CYP3A4 are primarily responsible for the conversion of paracetamol to NAPQI. In the kidney, cyclooxygenases are the principal route by which paracetamol is converted to NAPQI.[70] Paracetamol overdose leads to the accumulation of NAPQI, which undergoes conjugation with glutathione. Conjugation depletes glutathione, a natural antioxidant. This in combination with direct cellular injury by NAPQI, leads to cell damage and death.[71]

Paracetamol hepatotoxicity is, by far, the most common cause of acute liver failure in both the United States and the United Kingdom.[15] [72] Paracetamol overdose results in more calls to poison control centers in the US than overdose of any other pharmacological substance.[73] Signs and symptoms of paracetamol toxicity may initially be absent or vague. Untreated, overdose can lead to liver failure and death within days. Treatment is aimed at removing the paracetamol from the body and replacing glutathione. Activated charcoal can be used to decrease absorption of paracetamol if the patient presents for treatment soon after the overdose. While the antidote, acetylcysteine, (also called N-acetylcysteine or NAC) acts as a precursor for glutathione helping the body regenerate enough to prevent damage to the liver, a liver transplant is often required if damage to the liver becomes severe.[12]

In June 2009 an FDA advisory committee recommended that new restrictions should be placed on paracetamol to help protect people from the potential toxic effects.[74] [75]

Effects on animals

Paracetamol is extremely toxic to cats, and should not be given to them under any circumstances. Cats lack the necessary glucuronyl transferase enzymes to safely break paracetamol down, and minute portions of a tablet may prove fatal. Initial symptoms include vomiting, salivation and discolouration of the tongue and gums. Unlike an overdose in humans, liver damage is rarely the cause of death; instead, methaemoglobin formation and the production of Heinz bodies in red blood cells inhibit oxygen transport by the blood, causing asphyxiation (methemoglobemia and hemolytic anemia).[76] Treatment with N-acetylcysteine, methylene blue or both is sometimes effective after the ingestion of small doses of paracetamol. According to one paper female cats may have a better survival rate although sample size was small.[77]

Although paracetamol is believed to have no significant anti-inflammatory activity, it has been reported to be as effective as aspirin in the treatment of musculoskeletal pain in dogs.[78] A paracetamol-codeine product (trade name Pardale-V)[79] licensed for use in dogs is available on veterinary prescription in the UK.[80] It should be administered to dogs only on veterinary advice. The main effects of toxicity in dogs is liver damage.[81] N-acetylcysteine treatment is efficacious in dogs when administered within a few hours of paracetamol ingestion.[78]

Paracetamol is also lethal to snakes, and has been suggested as chemical control program for the brown tree snake (*Boiga irregularis*) in Guam.[82]

External links

- Paracetamol at Chemsynthesis [83]
- Paracetamol Information Centre [84]
- The Julius Axelrod Papers [85]
- FDA: Safe Use of Over-the-Counter Pain Relievers/Fever Reducers [86]
- FDA: Consumer education on Pain Relievers/Fever Reducers [87]
- FDA: Consumer Update "Acetaminophen and Liver Injury: Q and A for Consumers" (link) [88]
- FDA: Consumer Update "Acetaminophen and Liver Injury: Q and A for Consumers" (PDF) [89]

References

[1] http://www.nlm.nih.gov/cgi/mesh/2009/MB_cgi?term=103-90-2&rn=1
[2] http://www.whocc.no/atc_ddd_index/?code=N02BE01
[3] http://pubchem.ncbi.nlm.nih.gov/summary/summary.cgi?cid=1983
[4] http://www.drugbank.ca/cgi-bin/show_drug.cgi?CARD=APRD00252
[5] http://www.chemspider.com/Chemical-Structure.1906
[6] http://www.emolecules.com/cgi-bin/search?t=ex&q=C1%3DCC%28%3DCC%3DC1NC%28C%29%3DO%29O
[7] http://pubchem.ncbi.nlm.nih.gov/search/?smarts=C1%3DCC%28%3DCC%3DC1NC%28C%29%3DO%29O
[8] http://www.accessdata.fda.gov/scripts/cder/drugsatfda/index.cfm?fuseaction=Search.SearchAction&SearchTerm=ACETAMINOPHEN&SearchType=BasicSearch
[9] http://en.wikipedia.org/w/index.php?&diff=cur&oldid=306792031
[10] *Control of Pain in Patients with Cancer* Sign Guidelines **40** Section 6 (http://www.sign.ac.uk/guidelines/fulltext/44/section6.html).
[11] http://www.drugs.com/acetaminophen.html

[12] Daly FF, Fountain JS, Murray L, Graudins A, Buckley NA (March 2008). "Guidelines for the management of paracetamol poisoning in Australia and New Zealand—explanation and elaboration. A consensus statement from clinical toxicologists consulting to the Australasian poisons information centres" (http://www.mja.com.au/public/issues/188_05_030308/dal10916_fm.html). *Med. J. Aust.* **188** (5): 296–301. PMID 18312195 (http://www.ncbi.nlm.nih.gov/pubmed/18312195). .

[13] Khashab M, Tector AJ, Kwo PY (March 2007). "Epidemiology of acute liver failure". *Curr Gastroenterol Rep* **9** (1): 66–73. doi:10.1007/s11894-008-0023-x (http://dx.doi.org/10.1007/s11894-008-0023-x). PMID 17335680 (http://www.ncbi.nlm.nih.gov/pubmed/17335680).

[14] Hawkins LC, Edwards JN,PI (2007). "Impact of restricting paracetamol pack sizes on paracetamol poisoning in the United Kingdom: a review of the literature". *Drug Saf* **30** (6): 465–79. doi: 10.2165/00002018-200730060-00002 (http://dx.doi.org/10.2165/00002018-200730060-00002). PMID 17536874 (http://www.ncbi.nlm.nih.gov/pubmed/17536874).

[15] Larson AM, Polson J, Fontana RJ, *et al.* (2005). "Acetaminophen-induced acute liver failure: results of a United States multicenter, prospective study". *Hepatology* **42** (6): 1364–72. doi: 10.1002/hep.20948 (http://dx.doi.org/10.1002/hep.20948). PMID 16317692 (http://www.ncbi.nlm.nih.gov/pubmed/16317692).

[16] Bertolini A, Ferrari A, Ottani A, Guerzoni S, Tacchi R, Leone S (2006). "Paracetamol: new vistas of an old drug". *CNS drug reviews* **12** (3–4): 250–75. doi: 10.1111/j.1527-3458.2006.00250.x (http://dx.doi.org/10.1111/j.1527-3458.2006.00250.x). PMID 17227290 (http://www.ncbi.nlm.nih.gov/pubmed/17227290).

[17] Bergman K, Müller L, Teigen SW (February 1996). "The genotoxicity and carcinogenicity of paracetamol: a regulatory (re)view". *Mutat Res* **349** (2): 263–88. doi: 10.1016/0027-5107(95)00185-9 (http://dx.doi.org/10.1016/0027-5107(95)00185-9). PMID 8600357 (http://www.ncbi.nlm.nih.gov/pubmed/8600357).

[18] Bradley, N (September 1996). "BMJ should use "paracetamol" instead of "acetaminophen" in its index". *BMJ* **313** (7058): 689.

[19] Cahn, A; Hepp P. (1886). "Das Antifebrin, ein neues Fiebermittel". *Centralbl. Klin. Med.* **7**: 561–64.

[20] H. N. Morse (1878). "Ueber eine neue Darstellungsmethode der Acetylamidophenole". *Berichte der deutschen chemischen Gesellschaft* **11** (1): 232–233. doi: 10.1002/cber.18780110151 (http://dx.doi.org/10.1002/cber.18780110151).

[21] Milton Silverman, Mia Lydecker, Philip Randolph Lee (1992). *Bad Medicine: The Prescription Drug Industry in the Third World*. Stanford University Press. pp. 88–90. ISBN 0804716692.

[22] Von Mering J. Beitrage zur Kenntniss der Antipyretica. Ther Monatsch 1893;7:577–587.

[23] Sneader, Walter (2005). *Drug Discovery: A History*. Hoboken, N.J.: Wiley. p. 439. ISBN 0471899801.

[24] Lester D, Greenberg LA, Carroll RP (1947). "The metabolic fate of acetanilid and other aniline derivatives: II. Major metabolites of acetanilid appearing in the blood" (http://jpet.aspetjournals.org/cgi/reprint/90/1/68). *J. Pharmacol. Exp. Ther.* **90**: 68–75. .

[25] Brodie, BB; Axelrod J (1948). "The estimation of acetanilide and its metabolic products, aniline, *N*-acetyl *p*-aminophenol and *p*-aminophenol (free and total conjugated) in biological fluids and tissues". *J. Pharmacol. Exp. Ther.* **94** (1): 22–28. PMID 18885610 (http://www.ncbi.nlm.nih.gov/pubmed/18885610).

[26] Brodie, BB; Axelrod J (1948). "The fate of acetanilide in man" (http://profiles.nlm.nih.gov/HH/A/A/A/D/_/hhaaad.pdf) (PDF). *J. Pharmacol. Exp. Ther.* **94** (1): 29–38. PMID 18885611 (http://www.ncbi.nlm.nih.gov/pubmed/18885611). .

[27] Flinn, Frederick B; Brodie BB (1948). "The effect on the pain threshold of *N*-acetyl *p*-aminophenol, a product derived in the body from acetanilide". *J. Pharmacol. Exp. Ther.* **94** (1): 76–77. PMID 18885618 (http://www.ncbi.nlm.nih.gov/pubmed/18885618)..

[28] Brodie BB, Axelrod J (1949). "The fate of acetophenetidin (phenacetin) in man and methods for the estimation of acetophenitidin and its metabolites in biological material". *J Pharmacol Exp Ther* **94** (1): 58–67.

[29] " A Festival of Analgesics (http://www.chemheritage.org/EducationalServices/pharm/asp/asp08.htm)." *Chemical Heritage Foundation* (http://www.chemheritage.org/). 2001. Retrieved on August 17, 2007.

[30] US patent 6126967 (http://v3.espacenet.com/textdoc?DB=EPODOC&IDX=US6126967), *"Extended release acetaminophen particles"*, granted 2000-10-03

[31] Bales, JR; Nicholson JK, Sadler PJ (May 1, 1985). "Two-dimensional proton nuclear magnetic resonance "maps" of acetaminophen metabolites in human urine" (http://www.clinchem.org/cgi/reprint/31/5/757). *Clinical Chemistry* **31** (5): 757–762. PMID 3987005 (http://www.ncbi.nlm.nih.gov/pubmed/3987005). .

[32] Anthony S. Travis (2007). "Manufacture and uses of the anilines: A vast array of processes and products". in Zvi Rappoport. *The chemistry of Anilines Part 1*. Wiley. pp. 764. ISBN 978-0-470-87171-3.

[33] Bhattacharya A.; Purohit V. C.; Suarez, V.; Tichkule, R; Parmer, G.; Rinaldi, F. (2006). "One-step reductive amidation of nitro arenes: application in the synthesis of Acetaminophen". *Tetrahedron Letters* **47** (11): 1861–1864. doi: 10.1016/j.tetlet.2005.09.196 (http://dx.doi.org/10.1016/j.tetlet.2005.09.196).

[34] Ellis, Frank (2002). *Paracetamol: a curriculum resource*. Cambridge: Royal Society of Chemistry. ISBN 0-85404-375-6.

[35] Henney, K; Dudley B (1939). *Handbook of Photography*. Whittlesey House. pp. 324.

[36] "Acetaminophen." Physicians' Desk Reference, 63rd ed. Montvale, NJ: Thomson PDR; 2009:1915-1916.

[37] *Reader's Digest Guide to Drugs and Supplements*. Pleasantville, New York; Montreal: Reader's Digest Association, Inc.. 2002. ISBN 0-7621-0366-3.

[38] Rossi, S. (ed.) (2008). *Australian Medicines Handbook 2008* (http://www.amh.net.au). Adelaide: Australian Medicines Handbook. ISBN 0-9757919-6-7. .

[39] Kis B, Snipes JA, Busija DW (2005). "Acetaminophen and the cyclooxygenase-3 puzzle: sorting out facts, fictions, and uncertainties". *J. Pharmacol. Exp. Ther.* **315** (1): 1–7. doi: 10.1124/jpet.105.085431 (http://dx.doi.org/10.1124/jpet.105.085431). PMID 15879007 (http://

www.ncbi.nlm.nih.gov/pubmed/15879007).

[40] Aronoff DM, Oates JA, Boutaud O (2006). "New insights into the mechanism of action of acetaminophen: Its clinical pharmacologic characteristics reflect its inhibition of the two prostaglandin H2 synthases". *Clin. Pharmacol. Ther.* **79** (1): 9–19. doi: 10.1016/j.clpt.2005.09.009 (http://dx.doi.org/10.1016/j.clpt.2005.09.009). PMID 16413237 (http://www.ncbi.nlm.nih.gov/pubmed/16413237).

[41] Graham GG, Scott KF (2005). "Mechanism of action of paracetamol". *American journal of therapeutics* **12** (1): 46–55. doi: 10.1097/00045391-200501000-00008 (http://dx.doi.org/10.1097/00045391-200501000-00008). PMID 15662292 (http://www.ncbi.nlm.nih.gov/pubmed/15662292).

[42] Ohki S, Ogino N, Yamamoto S, Hayaishi O (1979). "Prostaglandin hydroperoxidase, an integral part of prostaglandin endoperoxide synthetase from bovine vesicular gland microsomes". *J. Biol. Chem.* **254** (3): 829–36. PMID 104998 (http://www.ncbi.nlm.nih.gov/pubmed/104998).

[43] Harvison PJ, Egan RW, Gale PH, Nelson SD (1986). "Acetaminophen as a cosubstrate and inhibitor of prostaglandin H synthase". *Adv. Exp. Med. Biol.* **197**: 739–47. PMID 3094341 (http://www.ncbi.nlm.nih.gov/pubmed/3094341).

[44] Roberts, LJ II. & Marrow, J.D. "Analgesic-antipyretic and Antiinflammatory Agents and Drugs Employed in the Treatment of Gout" in, "Goodman & Gilman's The Pharmacological Basis of Therapeutics 10th Edition" by Hardman, J.G. & Limbird, L.E. Published by McGraw Hill, 2001, p.687–731.

[45] Dinarello, Charles A.; Porat (2008). "Fever and Hyperthermia" (http://www.mhprofessional.com/product.php?isbn=0071466339&cat=4). in Kasper, Dennis L.; Braunwald, Eugene; Jameson, J. Larry et al.. *Harrison's Principles of Internal Medicine* (17th ed.). New York: McGraw-Hill Medical Publishing Division. ISBN 978-0-07-146633-9. .

[46] Högestätt ED, Jönsson BA, Ermund A, et al. (2005). "Conversion of acetaminophen to the bioactive N-acylphenolamine AM404 via fatty acid amide hydrolase-dependent arachidonic acid conjugation in the nervous system". *J. Biol. Chem.* **280** (36): 31405–12. doi: 10.1074/jbc.M501489200 (http://dx.doi.org/10.1074/jbc.M501489200). PMID 15987694 (http://www.ncbi.nlm.nih.gov/pubmed/15987694).

[47] Köfalvi A (2008). *Chapter 9: Alternative interacting sites and novel receptors for cannabinoid ligands. In: 'Cannabinoids and the Brain'* Springer-Verlag. pp. 131–160. doi: 10.1007/978-0-387-74349-3_9 (http://dx.doi.org/10.1007/978-0-387-74349-3_9).

[48] Ottani A, Leone S, Sandrini M, Ferrari A, Bertolini A (2006). "The analgesic activity of paracetamol is prevented by the blockade of cannabinoid CB1 receptors". *Eur. J. Pharmacol.* **531** (1–3): 280–1. doi: 10.1016/j.ejphar.2005.12.015 (http://dx.doi.org/10.1016/j.ejphar.2005.12.015). PMID 16438952 (http://www.ncbi.nlm.nih.gov/pubmed/16438952).

[49] Chandrasekharan NV, Dai H, Roos KL, et al. (2002). "COX-3, a cyclooxygenase-1 variant inhibited by acetaminophen and other analgesic/antipyretic drugs: cloning, structure, and expression" (http://www.pubmedcentral.nih.gov/articlerender.fcgi?tool=pmcentrez&artid=129799). *Proc. Natl. Acad. Sci. U.S.A.* **99** (21): 13926–31. doi: 10.1073/pnas.162468699 (http://dx.doi.org/10.1073/pnas.162468699). PMID 12242329 (http://www.ncbi.nlm.nih.gov/pubmed/12242329).

[50] Hendrickson, Robert G.; Kenneth E. Bizovi (2006). " Acetaminophen (http://books.google.com/books?id=cvJuLqBxGUcC&pg=PA525)", in Nelson, Lewis H.; Flomenbaum, Neal; Goldfrank, Lewis R. et al. *Goldfrank's toxicologic emergencies*, p. 525, New York: McGraw-Hill. Retrieved on January 18, 2009 through Google Book Search.

[51] Borne, Ronald F. "Nonsteroidal Anti-inflammatory Drugs" in *Principles of Medicinal Chemistry*, Fourth Edition. Eds. Foye, William O.; Lemke, Thomas L.; Williams, David A. Published by Williams & Wilkins, 1995. p. 544–545.

[52] Dong H, Haining RL, Thummel KE, Rettie AE, Nelson SD (2000). "Involvement of human cytochrome P450 2D6 in the bioactivation of acetaminophen". *Drug Metab Dispos* **28** (12): 1397–400. PMID 11095574 (http://www.ncbi.nlm.nih.gov/pubmed/11095574). Free full text (http://dmd.aspetjournals.org/cgi/content/full/28/12/1397)

[53] "Baby paracetamol asthma concern" (http://news.bbc.co.uk/1/hi/health/7623230.stm). BBC News. 2008-09-19. . Retrieved 2008-09-19.

[54] Bradley JD, Brandt KD, Katz BP, Kalasinski LA, Ryan SI (1991). "Comparison of an antiinflammatory dose of ibuprofen, an analgesic dose of ibuprofen, and acetaminophen in the treatment of patients with osteoarthritis of the knee". *N. Engl. J. Med.* **325** (2): 87–91. PMID 2052056 (http://www.ncbi.nlm.nih.gov/pubmed/2052056).

[55] doi: 10.1111/j.1365-2710.2006.00754.x (http://dx.doi.org/10.1111/j.1365-2710.2006.00754.x)

[56] Clark E, Plint AC, Correll R, Gaboury I, Passi B (2007). "A randomized, controlled trial of acetaminophen, ibuprofen, and codeine for acute pain relief in children with musculoskeletal trauma". *Pediatrics* **119** (3): 460–7. doi: 10.1542/peds.2006-1347 (http://dx.doi.org/10.1542/peds.2006-1347). PMID 17332198 (http://www.ncbi.nlm.nih.gov/pubmed/17332198).

[57] García Rodríguez LA, Hernández-Díaz S (December 15, 2000). "The risk of upper gastrointestinal complications associated with nonsteroidal anti-inflammatory drugs, glucocorticoids, acetaminophen, and combinations of these agents" (http://www.pubmedcentral.nih.gov/articlerender.fcgi?tool=pmcentrez&artid=128885). *Arthritis Research and Therapy* **3** (2): 98. doi: 10.1186/ar146 (http://dx.doi.org/10.1186/ar146). PMID 11178116 (http://www.ncbi.nlm.nih.gov/pubmed/11178116).

[58] http://news.bbc.co.uk/2/hi/health/3271191.stm

[59] Rudolph AM (February 1981). "Effects of aspirin and acetaminophen in pregnancy and in the newborn". *Arch. Intern. Med.* **141** (3 Spec No): 358–63. doi: 10.1001/archinte.141.3.358 (http://dx.doi.org/10.1001/archinte.141.3.358). PMID 7469626 (http://www.ncbi.nlm.nih.gov/pubmed/7469626).

[60] Lesko SM, Mitchell AA (October 1999). "The safety of acetaminophen and ibuprofen among children younger than two years old" (http://pediatrics.aappublications.org/cgi/pmidlookup?view=long&pmid=10506264). *Pediatrics* **104** (4): e39. doi: 10.1542/peds.104.4.e39 (http://

dx.doi.org/10.1542/peds.104.4.e39). PMID 10506264 (http://www.ncbi.nlm.nih.gov/pubmed/10506264). .

[61] Beasley, Richard; Clayton, Tadd; Crane, Julian; von Mutius, Erika; Lai, Christopher; Montefort, Stephen; Stewart, Alistair (2008). "Association between paracetamol use in infancy and childhood, and risk of asthma, rhino conjunctivitis, and eczema in children aged 6–7 years: analysis from Phase Three of the ISAAC programme." (http://www.thelancet.com/journals/lancet/article/PIIS0140673608614452/abstract). *The Lancet* **372**: 1039–1048. doi: 10.1016/S0140-6736(08)61445-2 (http://dx.doi.org/10.1016/S0140-6736(08)61445-2). . Retrieved 2008-09-19.

[62] The Lancet (2008). "Asthma: still more questions than answers". *The Lancet* **372**: 1009–1009. doi: 10.1016/S0140-6736(08)61414-2 (http://dx.doi.org/10.1016/S0140-6736(08)61414-2).

[63] Barr, R. G. (2008). "Does paracetamol cause asthma in children? Time to remove the guesswork". *The Lancet* **372**: 1011–1012. doi: 10.1016/S0140-6736(08)61417-8 (http://dx.doi.org/10.1016/S0140-6736(08)61417-8).

[64] Lawyer, A. B. (2009). "Paracetamol as a risk factor for allergic disorders". *The Lancet* **373**: 121–121. doi: 10.1016/S0140-6736(09)60032-5 (http://dx.doi.org/10.1016/S0140-6736(09)60032-5).

[65] Lowe, A. (2009). "Paracetamol as a risk factor for allergic disorders". *The Lancet* **373**: 120–120. doi: 10.1016/S0140-6736(09)60030-1 (http://dx.doi.org/10.1016/S0140-6736(09)60030-1).

[66] Lawrence, J. (2009). "Paracetamol as a risk factor for allergic disorders". *The Lancet* **373**: 119–119. doi: 10.1016/S0140-6736(09)60029-5 (http://dx.doi.org/10.1016/S0140-6736(09)60029-5).

[67] Singh, M. (2009). "Paracetamol as a risk factor for allergic disorders". *The Lancet* **373**: 119–119. doi: 10.1016/S0140-6736(09)60028-3 (http://dx.doi.org/10.1016/S0140-6736(09)60028-3).

[68] Beasley, R. (2009). "Paracetamol as a risk factor for allergic disorders – Authors' reply". *The Lancet* **373**: 120–121. doi: 10.1016/S0140-6736(09)60031-3 (http://dx.doi.org/10.1016/S0140-6736(09)60031-3).

[69] Medicines and Healthcare products Regulatory Agency; Commission on Human Medicines (2008). "Paracetamol use in infancy: no strong evidence for asthma link" (http://www.mhra.gov.uk/Publications/Safetyguidance/DrugSafetyUpdate/CON030923). *Drug Safety Update* **2** (4): 9. . Retrieved 2009-05-01.

[70] Mohandas J, Duggin GG, Horvath JS, Tiller DJ (November 1981). "Metabolic oxidation of acetaminophen (paracetamol) mediated by cytochrome P-450 mixed-function oxidase and prostaglandin endoperoxide synthetase in rabbit kidney" (http://linkinghub.elsevier.com/retrieve/pii/0041-008X(81)90415-4). *Toxicol. Appl. Pharmacol.* **61** (2): 252–9. doi: 10.1016/0041-008X(81)90415-4 (http://dx.doi.org/10.1016/0041-008X(81)90415-4). PMID 6798713 (http://www.ncbi.nlm.nih.gov/pubmed/6798713). .

[71] Mitchell JR, Jollow DJ, Potter WZ, Gillette JR, Brodie BB (October 1973). "Acetaminophen-induced hepatic necrosis. IV. Protective role of glutathione" (http://jpet.aspetjournals.org/cgi/pmidlookup?view=long&pmid=4746329). *The Journal of pharmacology and experimental therapeutics* **187** (1): 211–7. PMID 4746329 (http://www.ncbi.nlm.nih.gov/pubmed/4746329). .

[72] Ryder SD, Beckingham IJ (2001). "ABC of diseases of liver, pancreas, and biliary system. Other causes of parenchymal liver disease" (http://www.pubmedcentral.nih.gov/articlerender.fcgi?tool=pmcentrez&artid=1119531). *BMJ* **322** (7281): 290–92. doi: 10.1136/bmj.322.7281.290 (http://dx.doi.org/10.1136/bmj.322.7281.290). PMID 11157536 (http://www.ncbi.nlm.nih.gov/pubmed/11157536). [11157536 Free full text]

[73] Lee WM (July 2004). "Acetaminophen and the U.S. Acute Liver Failure Study Group: lowering the risks of hepatic failure" (http://www3.interscience.wiley.com/cgi-bin/fulltext/109086434/PDFSTART). *Hepatology* **40** (1): 6–9. doi: 10.1002/hep.20293 (http://dx.doi.org/10.1002/hep.20293). PMID 15239078 (http://www.ncbi.nlm.nih.gov/pubmed/15239078). .

[74] "FDA May Restrict Acetaminophen" (http://www.webmd.com/pain-management/news/20090701/fda-may-restrict-acetaminophen)

[75] "FDA: Drug Safety & Availability - Acetaminophen Information" (http://www.fda.gov/Drugs/DrugSafety/InformationbyDrugClass/ucm165107.htm)

[76] Allen AL (2003). "The diagnosis of acetaminophen toxicosis in a cat" (http://www.pubmedcentral.nih.gov/articlerender.fcgi?tool=pmcentrez&artid=340185). *Can Vet J* **44** (6): 509–10. PMID 12839249 (http://www.ncbi.nlm.nih.gov/pubmed/12839249).

[77] Rumbeiha WK, Lin YS, Oehme FW (November 1995). "Comparison of N-acetylcysteine and methylene blue, alone or in combination, for treatment of acetaminophen toxicosis in cats". *Am. J. Vet. Res.* **56** (11): 1529–33. PMID 8585668 (http://www.ncbi.nlm.nih.gov/pubmed/8585668).

[78] Maddison, Jill E.; Stephen W. Page, David Church (2002). *Small Animal Clinical Pharmacology*. Elsevier Health Sciences. pp. 260–261. ISBN 0702025739.

[79] "Pardale-V Tablets: Presentation" (http://www.noahcompendium.co.uk/Dechra/Pardale-V_Oral_Tablets/-27619.html). UK National Office of Animal Health Compendium of Animal Medicines. September 28, 2006. . Retrieved 3 January 2007.

[80] "Pardale-V Tablets: Legal Category" (http://www.noahcompendium.co.uk/Dechra/Pardale-V_Oral_Tablets/-27624.html). UK National Office of Animal Health Compendium of Animal Medicines. November 15, 2005. . Retrieved 3 January 2007.

[81] Villar D, Buck WB, Gonzalez JM (1998). "Ibuprofen, aspirin and acetaminophen toxicosis and treatment in dogs and cats". *Vet Hum Toxicol* **40** (3): 156–62. PMID 9610496 (http://www.ncbi.nlm.nih.gov/pubmed/9610496).

[82] Johnston J, Savarie P, Primus T, Eisemann J, Hurley J, Kohler D (2002). "Risk assessment of an acetaminophen baiting program for chemical control of brown tree snakes on Guam: evaluation of baits, snake residues, and potential primary and secondary hazards". *Environ Sci Technol* **36** (17): 3827–33. doi: 10.1021/es015873n (http://dx.doi.org/10.1021/es015873n). PMID 12322757 (http://www.ncbi.nlm.nih.gov/pubmed/12322757).

[83] http://www.chemsynthesis.com/base/chemical-structure-18651.html

[84] http://www.pharmweb.net/pwmirror/pwy/paracetamol/pharmwebpic.html

[85] http://profiles.nlm.nih.gov/HH/Views/Exhibit/narrative/amines.html
[86] http://www.fda.gov/Drugs/ResourcesForYou/Consumers/BuyingUsingMedicineSafely/UnderstandingOver-the-CounterMedicines/SafeUseofOver-the-CounterPainRelieversandFeverReducers/ucm164977.htm
[87] http://web.archive.org/web/20071217222733/www.fda.gov/usemedicinesafely/otc_text.htm
[88] http://www.fda.gov/ForConsumers/ConsumerUpdates/ucm168830.htm
[89] http://www.fda.gov/downloads/ForConsumers/ConsumerUpdates/UCM172664.pdf

Ibuprofen

1 : 1 mixture (racemate)

Systematic (IUPAC) name	
(RS)-2-(4-(2-methylpropyl)phenyl)propanoic acid	
Identifiers	
CAS number	15687-27-1 [1]
ATC code	M01 AE01 [2]
PubChem	3672 [3]
DrugBank	APRD00372 [4]
ChemSpider	3544 [5]
Chemical data	
Formula	$C_{13}H_{18}O_2$
Mol. mass	206.28
SMILES	eMolecules [6] & PubChem [7]
Physical data	
Melt. point	76 °C (169 °F)
Pharmacokinetic data	
Bioavailability	49–73%
Protein binding	99%
Metabolism	Hepatic (CYP2C9)
Half life	1.8–2 hours
Excretion	Renal
Therapeutic considerations	
Licence data	US FDA: link [8]
Pregnancy cat.	C(AU) D(US)
Legal status	Unscheduled (AU) GSL (UK) OTC (US)
Routes	Oral, rectal, topical, and intravenous
✓ (what is this?) (verify) [9]	

Ibuprofen (INN) (pronounced /ˈaɪbjuːproʊfɛn/ or /aɪbjuːˈproʊfən/; from the now outdated nomenclature iso-**bu**tyl-**pro**panoic-**phen**olic acid) is a non-steroidal anti-inflammatory drug (NSAID) originally marketed as **Brufen**, and since then under various other trademarks (see tradenames section), most notably Nurofen, Advil and Motrin. It is used for relief of symptoms of arthritis, primary dysmenorrhea, fever, and as an analgesic, especially where there is an inflammatory component. Ibuprofen is known to have an antiplatelet effect, though it is relatively mild and short-lived when compared with that of aspirin or other better-known antiplatelet drugs. Ibuprofen is a *core* medicine in the World Health Organization's "Essential Drugs List", which is a list of minimum medical needs for a basic health care system.[10]

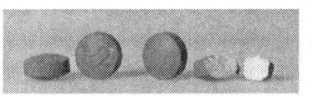

Coated 200 mg ibuprofen tablets

History

Ibuprofen was derived from propionic acid by the research arm of Boots Group during the 1960s.[11] It was discovered by Andrew RM Dunlop, with colleagues Stewart Adams, John Nicholson, Jeff Wilson & Colin Burrows and was patented in 1961. The drug was launched as a treatment for rheumatoid arthritis in the United Kingdom in 1969, and in the United States in 1974. Dr. Adams initially tested his drug on a hangover. He was subsequently awarded an OBE in 1987. Boots was awarded the Queen's Award For Technical Achievement for the development of the drug in 1987.[12]

2010 medication recall

On 15 January 2010, Johnson & Johnson announced the recall of several hundred batches of popular medicines, including Benadryl, Motrin, Rolaids, Simply Sleep, St. Joseph Aspirin and Tylenol[13] . The recall was due to contamination with the chemical 2,4,6-tribromoanisole[14] . The full health effects of 2,4,6-tribromoanisole are not known. The recall came 20 months after McNeil first began receiving consumer complaints about moldy-smelling bottles of Tylenol Arthritis Relief caplets, according to a warning letter sent by the Food and Drug Administration.

Typical administration

Low doses of ibuprofen (200 mg, and sometimes 400 mg) are available over the counter (OTC) in most countries. Ibuprofen has a dose-dependent duration of action of approximately 4–8 hours, which is longer than suggested by its short half-life. The recommended dose varies with body mass and indication. Generally, the oral dose is 200–400 mg (5–10 mg/kg in children) every 4–6 hours, adding up to a usual daily dose of 800–1,200 mg. 1,200 mg is considered the maximum daily dose for over-the-counter use, though under medical direction, the maximum amount of ibuprofen for adults is 800 milligrams per dose or 3200 mg per day (4 maximum doses).

Unlike aspirin, which breaks down in solution, ibuprofen is stable, and thus ibuprofen can be available in topical gel form which is absorbed through the skin, and can be used for sports injuries, with less risk of gastrointestinal problems.[15]

Off-label and investigational use

Ibuprofen is sometimes used for the treatment of acne, because of its anti-inflammatory properties,[16] and has been sold in Japan in topical form for adult acne.[17]

As with other NSAIDs, ibuprofen may be useful in the treatment of severe orthostatic hypotension (low blood pressure when standing up).[18]

In some studies, ibuprofen showed superior results compared to a placebo in the prophylaxis of Alzheimer's disease, when given in low doses over a long time.[19] Further studies are needed to confirm the results before ibuprofen can be recommended for this indication.

Ibuprofen has been associated with a lower risk of Parkinson's disease, and may delay or prevent it. Aspirin, other NSAIDs, and paracetamol had no effect on the risk for Parkinson's.[20] Further research is warranted before recommending ibuprofen for this use.

Ibuprofen lysine

In Europe, Australia, and New Zealand, **ibuprofen lysine** (the lysine salt of ibuprofen, sometimes called "ibuprofen lysinate" even though the lysine is in cationic form) is licensed for treatment of the same conditions as ibuprofen. The lysine salt increases water solubility, allowing the medication to be administered intravenously.[21] Ibuprofen lysine has been shown to have a more rapid onset of action compared to acid ibuprofen.[22]

Ibuprofen lysine is indicated for closure of a patent ductus arteriosus in premature infants weighing between 500 and 1500 grams, who are no more than 32 weeks gestational age when usual medical management (e.g., fluid restriction, diuretics, respiratory support, etc.) is ineffective.[21] With regard to this indication, ibuprofen lysine is an effective alternative to intravenous indomethacin and may be advantageous in terms of renal function.[23]

Mechanism of action

Non-steroidal anti-inflammatory drugs such as ibuprofen work by inhibiting the enzyme cyclooxygenase (COX), which converts arachidonic acid to prostaglandin H_2 (PGH_2). PGH_2, in turn, is converted by other enzymes to several other prostaglandins (which are mediators of pain, inflammation, and fever) and to thromboxane A_2 (which stimulates platelet aggregation, leading to the formation of blood clots).

Like aspirin, indomethacin, and most other NSAIDs, ibuprofen is considered a non-selective COX inhibitor—that is, it inhibits two isoforms of cyclooxygenase, *COX-1* and *COX-2*. The analgesic, antipyretic, and anti-inflammatory activity of NSAIDs appears to be achieved mainly through inhibition of COX-2, whereas inhibition of COX-1 would be responsible for unwanted effects on platelet aggregation and the gastrointestinal tract.[24] However, the role of the individual COX isoforms in the analgesic, anti-inflammatory, and gastric damage effects of NSAIDs is uncertain and different compounds cause different degrees of analgesia and gastric damage.[25]

Adverse effects

Ibuprofen appears to have the lowest incidence of gastrointestinal adverse drug reactions (ADRs) of all the non-selective NSAIDs. However, this only holds true at lower doses of ibuprofen, so over-the-counter preparations of ibuprofen are generally labeled to advise a maximum daily dose of 1,200 mg.[26][27]

Common adverse effects include: nausea, dyspepsia, gastrointestinal ulceration/bleeding, raised liver enzymes, diarrhea, constipation, epistaxis, headache, dizziness, priapism, rash, salt and fluid retention, and hypertension.[28]

Infrequent adverse effects include: esophageal ulceration, heart failure, hyperkalemia, renal impairment, confusion, and bronchospasm.[28]

Photosensitivity

As with other NSAIDs, ibuprofen has been reported to be a photosensitising agent.[29] [30] However, this only rarely occurs with ibuprofen and it is considered to be a very weak photosensitising agent when compared with other members of the 2-arylpropionic acid class. This is because the ibuprofen molecule contains only a single phenyl moiety and no bond conjugation, resulting in a very weak chromophore system and a very weak absorption spectrum which does not reach into the solar spectrum.

Cardiovascular risk

Along with several other NSAIDs, ibuprofen has been implicated in elevating the risk of myocardial infarction (heart attack), particularly among those chronically using high doses.[31]

Risks in inflammatory bowel disease (IBD)

Ibuprofen should not be used regularly in individuals with inflammatory bowel disease due to its ability to cause gastric bleeding and form ulceration in the gastric lining. Pain relievers such as paracetemol/acetaminophen or drugs containing codeine (which slows down bowel activity) are safer methods than ibuprofen for pain relief in IBD. Ibuprofen is also known to cause worsening of IBD during times of a flare-up, thus should be avoided completely.

Human toxicology

Ibuprofen overdose has become common since it was licensed for over-the-counter use. There are many overdose experiences reported in the medical literature, although the frequency of life-threatening complications from ibuprofen overdose is low.[32] Human response in cases of overdose ranges from absence of symptoms to fatal outcome in spite of intensive care treatment. Most symptoms are an excess of the pharmacological action of ibuprofen and include abdominal pain, nausea, vomiting, drowsiness, dizziness, headache, tinnitus, and nystagmus. Rarely more severe symptoms such as gastrointestinal bleeding, seizures, metabolic acidosis, hyperkalaemia, hypotension, bradycardia, tachycardia, atrial fibrillation, coma, hepatic dysfunction, acute renal failure, cyanosis, respiratory depression, and cardiac arrest have been reported.[33] The severity of symptoms varies with the ingested dose and the time elapsed; however, individual sensitivity also plays an important role. Generally, the symptoms observed with an overdose of ibuprofen are similar to the symptoms caused by overdoses of other NSAIDs.

There is little correlation between severity of symptoms and measured ibuprofen plasma levels. Toxic effects are unlikely at doses below 100 mg/kg but can be severe above 400 mg/kg; (around 150 200mg tablets for an average man)[34] however, large doses do not indicate that the clinical course is likely to be lethal.[35] It is not possible to determine a precise lethal dose, as this may vary with age, weight, and concomitant diseases of the individual patient.

Therapy is largely symptomatic. In cases presenting early, gastric decontamination is recommended. This is achieved using activated charcoal; charcoal absorbs the drug before it can enter the systemic circulation. Gastric lavage is now rarely used, but can be considered if the amount ingested is potentially life threatening and it can be performed within 60 minutes of ingestion. Emesis is not recommended.[36] The majority of ibuprofen ingestions produce only mild effects and the management of overdose is straightforward. Standard measures to maintain normal urine output should be instituted and renal function monitored.[34] Since ibuprofen has acidic properties and is also excreted in the urine, forced alkaline diuresis is theoretically beneficial. However, due to the fact ibuprofen is highly protein bound in the blood, there is minimal renal excretion of unchanged drug. Forced alkaline diuresis is therefore of limited benefit.[37] Symptomatic therapy for hypotension, GI bleeding, acidosis, and renal toxicity may be indicated. Occasionally, close monitoring in an intensive care unit for several days is necessary. If a patient survives the acute intoxication, they will usually experience no late sequelae.

Chemistry

Ibuprofen is only very slightly soluble in water, less than 1 mg of ibuprofen dissolves in 1 ml water (< 1 mg/mL).[38] However, it is much more soluble in alcohol/water mixtures.

Stereochemistry

Ibuprofen, like other 2-arylpropionate derivatives (including ketoprofen, flurbiprofen, naproxen, *etc*), contains a stereocenter in the α-position of the propionate moiety. As such, there are two possible enantiomers of ibuprofen, with the potential for different biological effects and metabolism for each enantiomer.

Indeed it was found that (*S*)-(+)-ibuprofen (dexibuprofen) was the active form both *in vitro* and *in vivo*.

It was logical, then, that there was the potential for improving the selectivity and potency of ibuprofen formulations by marketing ibuprofen as a single-enantiomer product (as occurs with naproxen, another NSAID).

Further *in vivo* testing, however, revealed the existence of an isomerase (*2-arylpropionyl-CoA epimerase*) which converted (*R*)-ibuprofen to the active (*S*)-enantiomer.[39] [40] [41] Thus, due to the expense and futility that might be involved in making a pure enantiomer, most ibuprofen formulations currently marketed are racemic mixtures.

Synthesis

The synthesis of this compound is a popular case study in green chemistry. The original Boots synthesis of ibuprofen consisted of six steps, started with the Friedel-Crafts acetylation of isobutylbenzene. Reaction with ethyl chloroacetate (Darzens reaction) gave the α,β-epoxy ester, which was decarboxylated and hydrolyzed to the aldehyde. Reaction with hydroxylamine gave the oxime, converted to the nitrile, then hydrolyzed to the desired acid:[42]

An improved synthesis by BHC required only three steps. This improved synthesis won the Presidential Green Chemistry Challenge Greener Synthetic Pathways Award in 1997.[43] After a similar acetylation, hydrogenation with Raney nickel gave the alcohol, which underwent palladium-catalyzed carbonylation:[42]

Availability

Ibuprofen was made available under prescription in the United Kingdom in 1969, and in the United States in 1974. In the years since, the good tolerability profile along with extensive experience in the population, as well as in so-called Phase IV trials (post-approval studies), has resulted in the availability of small packages of ibuprofen over the counter in pharmacies worldwide, as well as in supermarkets and other general retailers.

North America

In the United States, the Food and Drug Administration approved ibuprofen for over the counter use in 1984.

In North America doses between 100 mg and 400 mg are available over the counter. The 600 mg and 800 mg form is only available in North America by prescription.

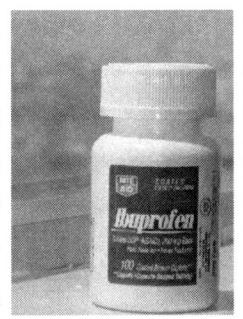

A bottle of generic ibuprofen

In 2009, the first injectable formulation of ibuprofen was approved in the United States, under the trade name *Caldolor*. Ibuprofen thus became the only parenteral for both pain and fever available in the country.[44]

Europe

For some time, there has been a limit on the amount that can be bought over the counter in a single transaction in the UK. Behind the counter in pharmacies this is one pack of 96 × 200 mg or 400 mg, the latter being far less common for over the counter sales. In UK non-pharmacy outlets only 200 mg tablets are allowed and they are restricted to a maximum pack of 16 tablets.

In Germany, 600 mg and 800 mg per pill packages have to be prescribed, whereas 400 mg is available over the counter in pharmacies. In Italy, Belgium and the Netherlands, 200 mg and 400 mg pills are available with no prescription.

In other countries, higher dosages of 600 mg are available.

External links

- U.S. National Library of Medicine: MedlinePlus Drug Information: Ibuprofen [45]
- University of Bristol chemistry department page on Ibuprofen [46]
- Nurofen UK Website [47]

References

[1] http://www.nlm.nih.gov/cgi/mesh/2009/MB_cgi?term=15687-27-1&rn=1
[2] http://www.whocc.no/atc_ddd_index/?code=M01AE01
[3] http://pubchem.ncbi.nlm.nih.gov/summary/summary.cgi?cid=3672
[4] http://www.drugbank.ca/cgi-bin/show_drug.cgi?CARD=APRD00372
[5] http://www.chemspider.com/Chemical-Structure.3544
[6] http://www.emolecules.com/cgi-bin/search?t=ex&q=CC%28C%28%3DO%29O%29c1ccc%28CC%28C%29C%29cc1
[7] http://pubchem.ncbi.nlm.nih.gov/search/?smarts=CC%28C%28%3DO%29O%29c1ccc%28CC%28C%29C%29cc1
[8] http://www.accessdata.fda.gov/scripts/cder/drugsatfda/index.cfm?fuseaction=Search.SearchAction&SearchTerm=Ibuprofen&SearchType=BasicSearch
[9] http://en.wikipedia.org/w/index.php?&diff=cur&oldid=307543575
[10] "WHO Model List of Essential Medicines" (http://whqlibdoc.who.int/hq/2005/a87017_eng.pdf) (PDF). World Health Organization. March 2005. . Retrieved 2006-03-12.
[11] Adams SS (April 1992). "The propionic acids: a personal perspective" (http://jcp.sagepub.com/cgi/reprint/32/4/317). *J Clin Pharmacol* **32** (4): 317–23. PMID 1569234 (http://www.ncbi.nlm.nih.gov/pubmed/1569234). .
[12] "Dr Stewart Adams: 'I tested ibuprofen on my hangover' - Telegraph" (http://www.telegraph.co.uk/health/main.jhtml?xml=/health/2007/10/08/hadams108.xml). . Retrieved 2008-01-20.
[13] In Recall, a Role Model Stumbles (http://www.nytimes.com/2010/01/18/business/18drug.html), Natasha Singer, New York Times, 17 January 2010.
[14] Tylenol recall expands (http://arthritis.webmd.com/news/20091229/tylenol-recall-expands), WebMD, accessed 1-17-2010.
[15] "Topical NSAIDs: plasma and tissue concentrations" (http://www.medicine.ox.ac.uk/bandolier/booth/painpag/topical/topkin.html). *Bandolier.* .
[16] RC, Wong; Kang S, Heezen JL, Voorhees JJ, Ellis CN. (Dec 1984). "Oral ibuprofen and tetracycline for the treatment of acne vulgaris." (http://www.ncbi.nlm.nih.gov/pubmed/6239884?ordinalpos=1&itool=EntrezSystem2.PEntrez.Pubmed.Pubmed_ResultsPanel.Pubmed_RVBrief). *Journal of the American Academy of Dermatology.* .
[17] "In Japan, an OTC ibuprofen ointment (Fukidia) for alleviating adult acne has been launched" (http://www.ingentaconnect.com/content/adis/inp/2006/00000001/00001530/art00048;jsessionid=1ghdlu0vup2pl.alice). *Inpharma* **1** (1530): 18. March 25, 2006. .
[18] Zawada, E. (1982). "Renal consequences of nonsteroidal antiinflammatory drugs". *Postgrad Med* **71** (5): 223–230. PMID 7041104 (http://www.ncbi.nlm.nih.gov/pubmed/7041104).
[19] Townsend KP, Praticò D (October 2005). "Novel therapeutic opportunities for Alzheimer's disease: focus on nonsteroidal anti-inflammatory drugs" (http://www.fasebj.org/cgi/content/full/19/12/1592). *FASEB J.* **19** (12): 1592–601. doi: 10.1096/fj.04-3620rev (http://dx.doi.org/10.1096/fj.04-3620rev). PMID 16195368 (http://www.ncbi.nlm.nih.gov/pubmed/16195368). . Retrieved 2008-12-08.
[20] Chen, H.; Jacobs, E.; Schwarzschild, M.; McCullough, M.; Calle, E.; Thun, M.; Ascherio, A. (2005). "Nonsteroidal antiinflammatory drug use and the risk for Parkinson's disease". *Ann Neurol* **58** (6): 963–967. doi: 10.1002/ana.20682 (http://dx.doi.org/10.1002/ana.20682). PMID 16240369 (http://www.ncbi.nlm.nih.gov/pubmed/16240369).
[21] Ovation Pharmaceuticals. "Neoprofen (ibuprofen lysine) injection". Package insert. (http://ovationpharma.com/pdfs/products/product_9.pdf)
[22] Geisslinger G, Dietzel K, Bezler H, Nuernberg B, Brune K (1989). "Therapeutically relevant differences in the pharmacokinetical and pharmaceutical behavior of ibuprofen lysinate as compared with ibuprofen acid.". *Int J Clin Pharmacol Ther Toxicol* **27** (7): 324–8. PMID 2777420 (http://www.ncbi.nlm.nih.gov/pubmed/2777420).
[23] Su PH, Chen JY, Su CM, Huang TC, Lee HS (2003). "Comparison of ibuprofen and indomethacin therapy for patent ductus arteriosus in preterm infants". *Pediatr Int* **45** (6): 665–70. doi: 10.1111/j.1442-200X.2003.01797.x (http://dx.doi.org/10.1111/j.1442-200X.2003.01797.x). PMID 14651538 (http://www.ncbi.nlm.nih.gov/pubmed/14651538).
[24] Rao P, Knaus EE (2008). "Evolution of nonsteroidal anti-inflammatory drugs (NSAIDs): cyclooxygenase (COX) inhibition and beyond" (https://ejournals.library.ualberta.ca/index.php/JPPS/article/viewFile/4128/3358). *J Pharm Pharm Sci* **11** (2): 81s–110s. PMID 19203472 (http://www.ncbi.nlm.nih.gov/pubmed/19203472). .
[25] Kakuta H, Zheng X, Oda H, et al. (April 2008). "Cyclooxygenase-1-selective inhibitors are attractive candidates for analgesics that do not cause gastric damage. design and in vitro/in vivo evaluation of a benzamide-type cyclooxygenase-1 selective inhibitor". *J. Med. Chem.* **51** (8): 2400–11. doi: 10.1021/jm701191z (http://dx.doi.org/10.1021/jm701191z). PMID 18363350 (http://www.ncbi.nlm.nih.gov/pubmed/18363350).
[26] "Ibuprofen - Drug information" (http://www.medic8.com/medicines/Ibuprofen.html). *Medic8.com.* .

[27] "Ibuprofen - Adverse effects" (http://www.experiencefestival.com/a/Ibuprofen_-_Adverse_effects/id/1494737). *Global Oneness.*.
[28] Rossi S, ed (2004). *Australian Medicines Handbook* (2004 ed.). Australian Medicines Handbook. ISBN 0-9578521-4-2. OCLC 224121065 (http://worldcat.org/oclc/224121065).
[29] Bergner T, Przybilla B. Photosensitization caused by ibuprofen. J Am Acad Dermatol 1992;26(1):114-6. PMID 1531054
[30] Thomson Healthcare. USP DI Advice for the Patient: Anti-inflammatory Drugs, Nonsteroidal (Systemic) [monograph on the internet]. Bethesda (MD): U.S. National Library of Medicine; c2006 [updated 2006 Jul 28; cited 2006 Aug 5]. Available from: http://www.nlm.nih.gov/medlineplus/druginfo/uspdi/202743.html
[31] Hippisley-Cox J, Coupland C (2005). "Risk of myocardial infarction in patients taking cyclo-oxygenase-2 inhibitors or conventional non-steroidal anti-inflammatory drugs: population based nested case-control analysis." (http://bmj.bmjjournals.com/cgi/content/full/330/7504/1366). *BMJ* **330** (7504): 1366. doi: 10.1136/bmj.330.7504.1366 (http://dx.doi.org/10.1136/bmj.330.7504.1366). PMID 15947398 (http://www.ncbi.nlm.nih.gov/pubmed/15947398). PMC 558288 (http://www.pubmedcentral.nih.gov/articlerender.fcgi?tool=pmcentrez&artid=558288). .
[32] McElwee NE, Veltri JC, Bradford DC, Rollins DE. (1990). "A prospective, population-based study of acute ibuprofen overdose: complications are rare and routine serum levels not warranted.". *Ann Emerg Med* **19** (6): 657–62. doi: 10.1016/S0196-0644(05)82471-0 (http://dx.doi.org/10.1016/S0196-0644(05)82471-0). PMID 2188537 (http://www.ncbi.nlm.nih.gov/pubmed/2188537).
[33] Vale JA, Meredith TJ. (1986). "Acute poisoning due to non-steroidal anti-inflammatory drugs. Clinical features and management.". *Med Toxicol* **1** (1): 12–31. PMID 3537613 (http://www.ncbi.nlm.nih.gov/pubmed/3537613).
[34] Volans G, Hartley V, McCrea S, Monaghan J. (2003). "Non-opioid analgesic poisoning". *Clinical Medicine* **3** (2): 119–23. doi: 10.1007/s10238-003-0014-z (http://dx.doi.org/10.1007/s10238-003-0014-z). PMID 12737366 (http://www.ncbi.nlm.nih.gov/pubmed/12737366).
[35] Seifert SA, Bronstein AC, McGuire T (2000). "Massive ibuprofen ingestion with survival". *J. Toxicol. Clin. Toxicol.* **38** (1): 55–7. doi: 10.1081/CLT-100100917 (http://dx.doi.org/10.1081/CLT-100100917). PMID 10696926 (http://www.ncbi.nlm.nih.gov/pubmed/10696926).
[36] American Academy Of Clinical Toxico; European Association Of Poisons Cen (2004). "Position paper: Ipecac syrup". *J. Toxicol. Clin. Toxicol.* **42** (2): 133–43. doi: 10.1081/CLT-120037421 (http://dx.doi.org/10.1081/CLT-120037421). PMID 15214617 (http://www.ncbi.nlm.nih.gov/pubmed/15214617).
[37] Hall AH, Smolinske SC, Conrad FL, *et al.* (1986). "Ibuprofen overdose: 126 cases". *Annals of emergency medicine* **15** (11): 1308–13. doi: 10.1016/S0196-0644(86)80617-5 (http://dx.doi.org/10.1016/S0196-0644(86)80617-5). PMID 3777588 (http://www.ncbi.nlm.nih.gov/pubmed/3777588).
[38] Motrin (Ibuprofen) drug description - FDA approved labeling for prescription drugs and medications at RxList (http://www.rxlist.com/cgi/generic/ibup.htm)
[39] Chen CS, Shieh WR, Lu PH, Harriman S, Chen CY (1991). "Metabolic stereoisomeric inversion of ibuprofen in mammals". *Biochim Biophys Acta* **1078** (3): 411–7. PMID 1859831 (http://www.ncbi.nlm.nih.gov/pubmed/1859831).
[40] Tracy TS, Hall SD (1992). "Metabolic inversion of (*R*)-ibuprofen. Epimerization and hydrolysis of ibuprofenyl-coenzyme A". *Drug Metab Dispos* **20** (2): 322–7. PMID 1352228 (http://www.ncbi.nlm.nih.gov/pubmed/1352228).
[41] Reichel C, Brugger R, Bang H, Geisslinger G, Brune K (1997). "Molecular cloning and expression of a 2-arylpropionyl-coenzyme A epimerase: a key enzyme in the inversion metabolism of ibuprofen". *Mol Pharmacol* **51** (4): 576–82. PMID 9106621 (http://www.ncbi.nlm.nih.gov/pubmed/9106621). Free full text (http://molpharm.aspetjournals.org/cgi/content/full/51/4/576)
[42] http://www.rsc.org/education/teachers/learnnet/green/ibuprofen/
[43] "Presidential Green Chemistry Challenge: 1997 Greener Synthetic Pathways Award" (http://www.epa.gov/greenchemistry/pubs/pgcc/winners/gspa97.html). U.S. Environmental Protection Agency. . Retrieved 2009-08-18.
[44] Drugs.com (June 11, 2009). "FDA Approves Caldolor: Cumberland Pharmaceuticals Announces FDA Approval of Caldolor" (http://www.drugs.com/newdrugs/cumberland-pharmaceuticals-announces-fda-approval-caldolor-1447.html). Press release. . Retrieved 2009-06-13.
[45] http://www.nlm.nih.gov/medlineplus/druginfo/meds/a682159.html
[46] http://www.chm.bris.ac.uk/motm/ibuprofen/homepage.htm
[47] http://www.nurofen.co.uk

Myocardial infarction

Myocardial infarction
Classification and external resources

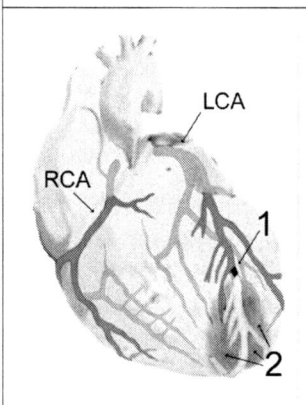

Diagram of a **myocardial infarction** (2) of the tip of the anterior wall of the heart (an *apical infarct*) after occlusion (1) of a branch of the left coronary artery (LCA, right coronary artery = RCA).

ICD-10	I 21.[1]-I 22.[2]
ICD-9	410 [3]
DiseasesDB	8664 [4]
MedlinePlus	000195 [5]
eMedicine	med/1567 [6] emerg/327 [7] ped/2520 [8]
MeSH	D009203 [9]

Myocardial infarction (MI) or **acute myocardial infarction (AMI)**, commonly known as a **heart attack**, is the interruption of blood supply to part of the heart, causing some heart cells to die. This is most commonly due to occlusion (blockage) of a coronary artery following the rupture of a vulnerable atherosclerotic plaque, which is an unstable collection of lipids (fatty acids) and white blood cells (especially macrophages) in the wall of an artery. The resulting ischemia (restriction in blood supply) and oxygen shortage, if left untreated for a sufficient period of time, can cause damage or death (*infarction*) of heart muscle tissue (*myocardium*).

Classical symptoms of acute myocardial infarction include sudden chest pain (typically radiating to the left arm or left side of the neck), shortness of breath, nausea, vomiting, palpitations, sweating, and anxiety (often described as a sense of impending doom). Women may experience fewer typical symptoms than men, most commonly shortness of breath, weakness, a feeling of indigestion, and fatigue.[10] Approximately one quarter of all myocardial infarctions are silent, without chest pain or other symptoms.

A heart attack is a medical emergency, and people experiencing chest pain are advised to alert their emergency medical services because prompt protection with an external defibrillator can save one's life from primary ventricular fibrillation which occurs unexpectedly in 10% of all myocardial infarctions especially during the first hours of symptoms. Contemporary treatment of many myocardial infarctions can result in survival and even good outcomes. While it is true that certain less amenable cases are very massive and rapidly fatal "widowmakers", it is also true that in small attacks with limited damage and optimal treatment the heart muscle can be salvaged.

Heart attacks are the leading cause of death for both men and women all over the world.[11] Important risk factors are previous cardiovascular disease (such as angina, a previous heart attack or stroke), older age (especially men over 40 and women over 50), tobacco smoking, high blood levels of certain lipids (triglycerides, low-density lipoprotein or "bad cholesterol") and low levels of high density lipoprotein (HDL, "good cholesterol"), diabetes, high blood pressure, obesity, chronic kidney disease, heart failure, excessive alcohol consumption, the abuse of certain drugs (such as cocaine and methamphetamine), and chronic high stress levels.[12] [13]

Immediate treatment for suspected acute myocardial infarction includes oxygen, aspirin, and sublingual glyceryl trinitrate (also known as nitroglycerin and abbreviated as NTG or GTN). Pain relief is also often given, classically morphine sulfate.[14] A 2009 review about the use of high flow oxygen for treating myocardial infarction found high flow oxygen administration increased mortality and infarct size, calling into question the recommendation for its routine use.[15]

The patient will receive a number of diagnostic tests, such as an electrocardiogram (ECG, EKG), a chest X-ray and blood tests to detect elevations in cardiac markers (blood tests to detect heart muscle damage). The most often used markers are the creatine kinase-MB (CK-MB) fraction and the troponin I (TnI) or troponin T (TnT) levels. On the basis of the ECG, a distinction is made between **ST elevation MI (STEMI)** or **non-ST elevation MI (NSTEMI** or **non-STEMI)**. Most cases of STEMI are treated with thrombolysis or if possible with percutaneous coronary intervention (PCI, angioplasty and stent insertion), provided the hospital has facilities for coronary angiography. NSTEMI is managed with medication, although PCI is often performed during hospital admission. In patients who have multiple blockages and who are relatively stable, or in a few extraordinary emergency cases, bypass surgery of the blocked coronary artery is an option.

The phrase "heart attack" is sometimes used incorrectly to describe sudden cardiac death, which may or may not be the result of acute myocardial infarction. A heart attack is different from, but can be the cause of cardiac arrest, which is the stopping of the heartbeat, and cardiac arrhythmia, an abnormal heartbeat. It is also distinct from heart failure, in which the pumping action of the heart is impaired; severe myocardial infarction may lead to heart failure, but not necessarily.

Classification

There are two basic types of acute myocardial infarction:
- Transmural: associated with atherosclerosis involving major coronary artery. It can be subclassified into anterior, posterior, or inferior. Transmural infarcts extend through the whole thickness of the heart muscle and are usually a result of complete occlusion of the area's blood supply.
- Subendocardial: involves small area in the subendocardial wall of the left ventricle, ventricular septum, or papillary muscles. Subendocardial infarcts are thought to be a result of locally decreased blood supply, possibly from a narrowing of the coronary arteries. The subendocardial area is farthest from the heart's blood supply and is more susceptible to this type of pathology.

Clinically, myocardial infarction is further subclassified into ST elevation MI versus non ST elevation MI based on ECG changes.

Signs and symptoms

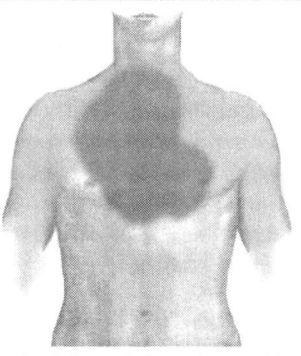

The onset of symptoms in myocardial infarction (MI) is usually gradual, over several minutes, and rarely instantaneous.[16] Chest pain is the most common symptom of acute myocardial infarction and is often described as a sensation of tightness, pressure, or squeezing. Chest pain due to ischemia (a lack of blood and hence oxygen supply) of the heart muscle is termed angina pectoris. Pain radiates most often to the left arm, but may also radiate to the lower jaw, neck, right arm, back, and epigastrium, where it may mimic heartburn. Levine's sign, in which the patient localizes the chest pain by clenching their fist over the sternum, has classically been thought to be predictive of cardiac chest pain, although a prospective observational study showed that it had a poor positive predictive value.[17]

Rough diagram of pain zones in myocardial infarction (dark red = most typical area, light red = other possible areas, view of the chest).

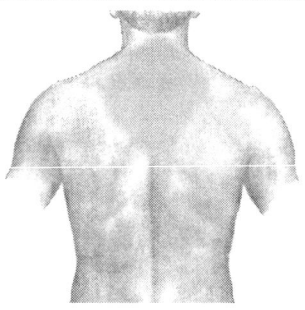

Shortness of breath (dyspnea) occurs when the damage to the heart limits the output of the left ventricle, causing left ventricular failure and consequent pulmonary edema. Other symptoms include diaphoresis (an excessive form of sweating), weakness, light-headedness, nausea, vomiting, and palpitations. These symptoms are likely induced by a massive surge of catecholamines from the sympathetic nervous system[18] which occurs in response to pain and the hemodynamic abnormalities that result from cardiac dysfunction. Loss of consciousness (due to inadequate cerebral perfusion and cardiogenic shock) and even sudden death (frequently due to the development of ventricular fibrillation) can occur in myocardial infarctions.

Women and older patients experience atypical symptoms more frequently than their male and younger counterparts.[19] Women also have more symptoms compared to men (2.6 on average vs 1.8 symptoms in men).[19] The most common symptoms of MI in women

Back view.

include dyspnea, weakness, and fatigue. Fatigue, sleep disturbances, and dyspnea have been reported as frequently occurring symptoms which may manifest as long as one month before the actual clinically manifested ischemic event. In women, chest pain may be less predictive of coronary ischemia than in men.[20]

Approximately half of all MI patients have experienced warning symptoms such as chest pain prior to the infarction.[21]

Approximately one fourth of all myocardial infarctions are silent, without chest pain or other symptoms.[22] These cases can be discovered later on electrocardiograms, using blood enzyme tests or at autopsy without a prior history of related complaints. A silent course is more common in the elderly, in patients with diabetes mellitus[23] and after heart transplantation, probably because the donor heart is not connected to nerves of the host.[24] In diabetics, differences in pain threshold, autonomic neuropathy, and psychological factors have been cited as possible explanations for the lack of symptoms.[23]

Any group of symptoms compatible with a sudden interruption of the blood flow to the heart are called an acute coronary syndrome.[25]

The differential diagnosis includes other catastrophic causes of chest pain, such as pulmonary embolism, aortic dissection, pericardial effusion causing cardiac tamponade, tension pneumothorax, and esophageal rupture.[26]

Causes and risk factors

Heart attack rates are higher in association with intense exertion, be it psychological stress or physical exertion, especially if the exertion is more intense than the individual usually performs.[27] Quantitatively, the period of intense exercise and subsequent recovery is associated with about a 6-fold higher myocardial infarction rate (compared with other more relaxed time frames) for people who are physically very fit.[27] For those in poor physical condition, the rate differential is over 35-fold higher.[27] One observed mechanism for this phenomenon is the increased arterial pulse pressure stretching and relaxation of arteries with each heart beat which, as has been observed with intravascular ultrasound, increases mechanical "shear stress" on atheromas and the likelihood of plaque rupture.[27]

Acute severe infection, such as pneumonia, can trigger myocardial infarction. A more controversial link is that between *Chlamydophila pneumoniae* infection and atherosclerosis.[28] While this intracellular organism has been demonstrated in atherosclerotic plaques, evidence is inconclusive as to whether it can be considered a causative factor.[28] Treatment with antibiotics in patients with proven atherosclerosis has not demonstrated a decreased risk of heart attacks or other coronary vascular diseases.[29]

There is an association of an increased incidence of a heart attack in the morning hours, more specifically around 9 a.m.[30] [31] [32]. Some investigators have noticed that the ability of platelets to aggregate varies according to a circadian rhythm, although they have not proven causation.[33] Some investigators theorize that this increased incidence may be related to the circadian variation in cortisol production affecting the concentrations of various cytokines and other mediators of inflammation.[34]

Risk factors

Risk factors for atherosclerosis are generally risk factors for myocardial infarction:

- Diabetes (with or without insulin resistance) - the single most important risk factor for ischaemic heart disease (IHD)
- Tobacco smoking
- Hypercholesterolemia (more accurately hyperlipoproteinemia, especially high low density lipoprotein and low high density lipoprotein)
- High blood pressure
- Family history of ischaemic heart disease (IHD)
- Obesity[35] (defined by a body mass index of more than 30 kg/m², or alternatively by waist circumference or waist-hip ratio).
- Age: Men acquire an independent risk factor at age 45, Women acquire an independent risk factor at age 55; in addition individuals acquire another independent risk factor if they have a first-degree male relative (brother, father) who suffered a coronary vascular event at or before age 55. Another independent risk factor is acquired if one has a first-degree female relative (mother, sister) who suffered a coronary vascular event at age 65 or younger.
- Hyperhomocysteinemia (high homocysteine, a toxic blood amino acid that is elevated when intakes of vitamins B2, B6, B12 and folic acid are insufficient)
- Stress (occupations with high stress index are known to have susceptibility for atherosclerosis)
- Alcohol Studies show that prolonged exposure to high quantities of alcohol can increase the risk of heart attack

Males are more at risk than females.[27]

Many of these risk factors are modifiable, so many heart attacks can be prevented by maintaining a healthier lifestyle. Physical activity, for example, is associated with a lower risk profile.[36] Non-modifiable risk factors include age, sex, and family history of an early heart attack (before the age of 60), which is thought of as reflecting a genetic predisposition.[27]

Socioeconomic factors such as a shorter education and lower income (particularly in women), and unmarried cohabitation may also contribute to the risk of MI.[37] To understand epidemiological study results, it's important to note that many factors associated with MI mediate their risk via other factors. For example, the effect of education is partially based on its effect on income and marital status.[37]

Women who use combined oral contraceptive pills have a modestly increased risk of myocardial infarction, especially in the presence of other risk factors, such as smoking.[38]

Inflammation is known to be an important step in the process of atherosclerotic plaque formation.[39] C-reactive protein (CRP) is a sensitive but non-specific marker for inflammation. Elevated CRP blood levels, especially measured with high sensitivity assays, can predict the risk of MI, as well as stroke and development of diabetes.[39] Moreover, some drugs for MI might also reduce CRP levels.[39] The use of high sensitivity CRP assays as a means of screening the general population is advised against, but it may be used optionally at the physician's discretion, in patients who already present with other risk factors or known coronary artery disease.[40] Whether CRP plays a direct role in atherosclerosis remains uncertain.[39]

Inflammation in periodontal disease may be linked coronary heart disease, and since periodontitis is very common, this could have great consequences for public health.[41] Serological studies measuring antibody levels against typical periodontitis-causing bacteria found that such antibodies were more present in subjects with coronary heart disease.[42] Periodontitis tends to increase blood levels of CRP, fibrinogen and cytokines;[43] thus, periodontitis may mediate its effect on MI risk via other risk factors.[44] Preclinical research suggests that periodontal bacteria can promote aggregation of platelets and promote the formation of foam cells.[45] [46] A role for specific periodontal bacteria has been suggested but remains to be established.[47] There is some evidence that influenza may trigger a acute myocardial infarction.[48]

Baldness, hair greying, a diagonal earlobe crease (Frank's sign[49]) and possibly other skin features have been suggested as independent risk factors for MI.[50] Their role remains controversial; a common denominator of these signs and the risk of MI is supposed, possibly genetic.[51]

Calcium deposition is another part of atherosclerotic plaque formation. Calcium deposits in the coronary arteries can be detected with CT scans. Several studies have shown that coronary calcium can provide predictive information beyond that of classical risk factors.[52] [53] [54]

The European Society of Cardiology and the European Association for Cardiovascular Prevention and Rehabilitation have developed an interactive tool for prediction and managing the risk of heart attack and stroke in Europe. HeartScore is aimed at supporting clinicians in optimising individual cardiovascular risk reduction. The Heartscore Programme is available in 12 languages and offers web based or PC version ([55]).

Pathophysiology

Acute myocardial infarction refers to two subtypes of acute coronary syndrome, namely **non-ST-elevated myocardial infarction** and **ST-elevated myocardial infarction**, which are most frequently (but not always) a manifestation of coronary artery disease. The most common triggering event is the disruption of an atherosclerotic plaque in an epicardial coronary artery, which leads to a clotting cascade, sometimes resulting in total occlusion of the artery. Atherosclerosis is the gradual buildup of cholesterol and fibrous tissue in plaques in the wall of arteries (in this case, the coronary arteries), typically over decades. Blood stream column irregularities visible on angiography reflect artery lumen narrowing as a result of decades of advancing atherosclerosis. Plaques can become unstable, rupture, and additionally promote a thrombus (blood clot) that occludes the artery; this can occur in minutes. When a severe enough plaque rupture occurs in the coronary vasculature, it leads to myocardial infarction (necrosis of downstream myocardium).

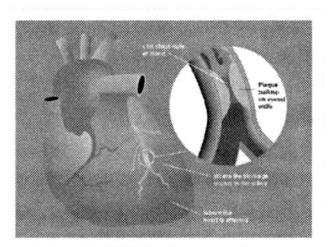

A myocardial infarction occurs when an atherosclerotic plaque slowly builds up in the inner lining of a coronary artery and then suddenly ruptures, totally occluding the artery and preventing blood flow downstream.

If impaired blood flow to the heart lasts long enough, it triggers a process called the ischemic cascade; the heart cells in the territory of the occluded coronary artery die (chiefly through necrosis) and do not grow back. A collagen scar forms in its place. Recent studies indicate that another form of cell death called apoptosis also plays a role in the process of tissue damage subsequent to myocardial infarction.[56] As a result, the patient's heart will be permanently damaged. This Myocardial scarring also puts the patient at risk for potentially life threatening arrhythmias, and may result in the formation of a ventricular aneurysm that can rupture with catastrophic consequences.

Injured heart tissue conducts electrical impulses more slowly than normal heart tissue. The difference in conduction velocity between injured and uninjured tissue can trigger re-entry or a feedback loop that is believed to be the cause of many lethal arrhythmias. The most serious of these arrhythmias is ventricular fibrillation (*V-Fib*/VF), an extremely fast and chaotic heart rhythm that is the leading cause of sudden cardiac death. Another life threatening arrhythmia is ventricular tachycardia (*V-Tach*/VT), which may or may not cause sudden cardiac death. However, ventricular tachycardia usually results in rapid heart rates that prevent the heart from pumping blood effectively. Cardiac output and blood pressure may fall to dangerous levels, which can lead to further coronary ischemia and extension of the infarct.

The cardiac defibrillator is a device that was specifically designed to terminate these potentially fatal arrhythmias. The device works by delivering an electrical shock to the patient in order to depolarize a critical mass of the heart muscle, in effect "rebooting" the heart. This therapy is time dependent, and the odds of successful defibrillation decline rapidly after the onset of cardiopulmonary arrest.

Diagnosis

The diagnosis of myocardial infarction is made by integrating the history of the presenting illness and physical examination with electrocardiogram findings and cardiac markers (blood tests for heart muscle cell damage).[57] A coronary angiogram allows visualization of narrowings or obstructions on the heart vessels, and therapeutic measures can follow immediately. At autopsy, a pathologist can diagnose a myocardial infarction based on anatomopathological findings.

A chest radiograph and routine blood tests may indicate complications or precipitating causes and are often performed upon arrival to an emergency department. New regional wall motion abnormalities on an echocardiogram are also suggestive of a myocardial infarction. Echo may be performed in equivocal cases by the on-call cardiologist.[58] In stable patients whose symptoms have resolved by the time of evaluation, Technetium (99mTc) sestamibi (i.e. a "MIBI scan") or thallium-201 chloride can be used in nuclear medicine to visualize areas of reduced blood flow in conjunction with physiologic or pharmocologic stress.[58] [59] Thallium may also be used to determine viability of tissue, distinguishing whether non-functional myocardium is actually dead or merely in a state of hibernation or of being stunned.[60]

Diagnostic criteria

WHO criteria[61] formulated in 1979 have classically been used to diagnose MI; a patient is diagnosed with myocardial infarction if two (probable) or three (definite) of the following criteria are satisfied:
1. Clinical history of ischaemic type chest pain lasting for more than 20 minutes
2. Changes in serial ECG tracings
3. Rise and fall of serum cardiac biomarkers such as creatine kinase-MB fraction and troponin

The WHO criteria were refined in 2000 to give more prominence to cardiac biomarkers.[62] According to the new guidelines, a cardiac troponin rise accompanied by either typical symptoms, pathological Q waves, ST elevation or depression or coronary intervention are diagnostic of MI.

Physical examination

The general appearance of patients may vary according to the experienced symptoms; the patient may be comfortable, or restless and in severe distress with an increased respiratory rate. A cool and pale skin is common and points to vasoconstriction. Some patients have low-grade fever (38–39 °C). Blood pressure may be elevated or decreased, and the pulse can be become irregular.[63] [64]

If heart failure ensues, elevated jugular venous pressure and hepatojugular reflux, or swelling of the legs due to peripheral edema may be found on inspection. Rarely, a cardiac bulge with a pace different from the pulse rhythm can be felt on precordial examination. Various abnormalities can be found on auscultation, such as a third and fourth heart sound, systolic murmurs, paradoxical splitting of the second heart sound, a pericardial friction rub and rales over the lung.[63] [64]

Electrocardiogram

The primary purpose of the electrocardiogram is to detect ischemia or acute coronary injury in broad, symptomatic emergency department populations. However, the standard 12 lead ECG has several limitations. An ECG represents a brief sample in time. Because unstable ischemic syndromes have rapidly changing supply versus demand characteristics, a single ECG may not accurately represent the entire picture.[65] It is therefore desirable to obtain *serial* 12 lead ECGs, particularly if the first ECG is obtained during a pain-free episode. Alternatively, many emergency departments and chest pain centers use computers capable of continuous ST segment monitoring.[66] The standard 12 lead ECG also does not directly examine the right ventricle, and is relatively poor at examining the posterior basal and lateral walls of the left ventricle. In particular, acute myocardial infarction in the distribution of the circumflex artery is likely to produce a nondiagnostic ECG.[65] The use of additional ECG leads like right-sided leads V3R and V4R and posterior leads V7, V8, and V9 may improve sensitivity for right ventricular and posterior myocardial infarction. In spite of these limitations, the 12 lead ECG stands at the center of risk stratification for the patient with suspected acute myocardial infarction. Mistakes in interpretation are relatively common, and the failure to identify high risk features has a negative effect on the quality of patient care.[67]

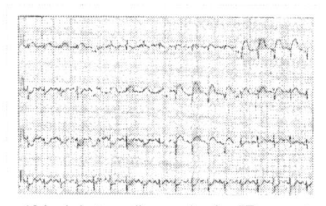

12-lead electrocardiogram showing ST-segment elevation (orange) in I, aVL and V1-V5 with reciprocal changes (blue) in the inferior leads, indicative of an anterior wall myocardial infarction.

The 12 lead ECG is used to classify patients into one of three groups:[68]
1. those with ST segment elevation or new bundle branch block (suspicious for acute injury and a possible candidate for acute reperfusion therapy with thrombolytics or primary PCI),
2. those with ST segment depression or T wave inversion (suspicious for ischemia), and
3. those with a so-called non-diagnostic or normal ECG.

A normal ECG does not rule out acute myocardial infarction. Sometimes the earliest presentation of acute myocardial infarction is the hyperacute T wave, which is treated the same as ST segment elevation.[69] In practice this is rarely seen, because it only exists for 2–30 minutes after the onset of infarction.[70] Hyperacute T waves need to be distinguished from the peaked T waves associated with hyperkalemia.[71] The current guidelines for the ECG diagnosis of acute myocardial infarction require at least 1 mm (0.1 mV) of ST segment elevation in the limb leads, and at least 2 mm elevation in the precordial leads. These elevations must be present in anatomically contiguous leads.[68] (I, aVL, V5, V6 correspond to the lateral wall; V1-V4 correspond to the anterior wall; II, III, aVF correspond to the inferior wall.) This criterion is problematic, however, as acute myocardial infarction is not the most common cause of ST segment elevation in chest pain patients.[72] Over 90% of healthy men have at least 1 mm (0.1 mV) of ST segment elevation in at least one precordial lead.[73] The clinician must therefore be well versed in recognizing the so-called ECG mimics of acute myocardial infarction, which include left ventricular hypertrophy, left bundle branch block, paced rhythm, early repolarization, pericarditis, hyperkalemia, and ventricular aneurysm.[73] [74] [75]

Cardiac markers

Cardiac markers or cardiac enzymes are proteins that leak out of injured myocardial cells through their damaged cell membranes into the bloodstream. Until the 1980s, the enzymes SGOT and LDH were used to assess cardiac injury. Now, the markers most widely used in detection of MI are *MB* subtype of the enzyme creatine kinase and cardiac troponins T and I as they are more specific for myocardial injury. The cardiac troponins T and I which are released within 4–6 hours of an attack of MI and remain elevated for up to 2 weeks, have nearly complete tissue specificity and are now the preferred markers for asssessing myocardial damage.[76] Elevated troponins in the setting of chest pain may accurately predict a high likelihood of a myocardial infarction in the near future.[77] New markers such as glycogen phosphorylase isoenzyme BB are under investigation.[78]

The diagnosis of myocardial infarction requires two out of three components (history, ECG, and enzymes). When damage to the heart occurs, levels of cardiac markers rise over time, which is why blood tests for them are taken over a 24-hour period. Because these enzyme levels are not elevated immediately following a heart attack, patients presenting with chest pain are generally treated with the assumption that a myocardial infarction has occurred and then evaluated for a more precise diagnosis.[79]

Angiography

In difficult cases or in situations where intervention to restore blood flow is appropriate, coronary angiography can be performed. A catheter is inserted into an artery (usually the femoral artery) and pushed to the vessels supplying the heart. A radio-opaque dye is administered through the catheter and a sequence of x-rays (fluoroscopy) is performed. Obstructed or narrowed arteries can be identified, and angioplasty applied as a therapeutic measure (see below). Angioplasty requires extensive skill, especially in emergency settings. It is performed by a physician trained in interventional cardiology.

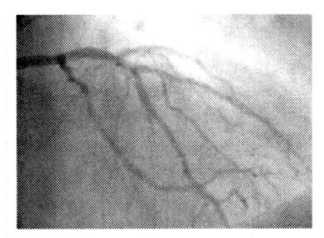

Angiogram of the coronary arteries.

Histopathology

Histopathological examination of the heart may reveal infarction at autopsy. Under the microscope, myocardial infarction presents as a circumscribed area of ischemic, coagulative necrosis (cell death). On gross examination, the infarct is not identifiable within the first 12 hours.[80]

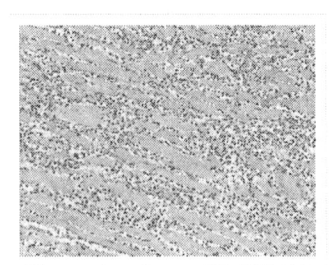

Microscopy image (magn. ca 100x, H&E stain) from autopsy specimen of myocardial infarct (7 days post-infarction).

Although earlier changes can be discerned using electron microscopy, one of the earliest changes under a normal microscope are so-called *wavy fibers*.[81] Subsequently, the myocyte cytoplasm becomes more eosinophilic (pink) and the cells lose their transversal striations, with typical changes and eventually loss of the cell nucleus.[82] The interstitium at the margin of the infarcted area is initially infiltrated with neutrophils, then with lymphocytes and macrophages, who phagocytose ("eat") the myocyte debris. The necrotic area is surrounded and progressively invaded by granulation tissue, which will replace the infarct with a fibrous (collagenous) scar (which are typical steps in wound healing). The interstitial space (the space between cells outside of blood vessels) may be infiltrated with red blood cells.[80]

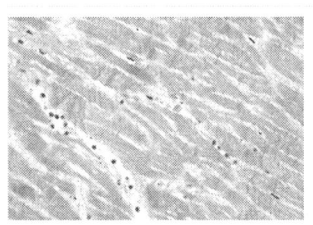

Micrograph of a **myocardial infarction** (ca. 400x H&E stain) with prominent contraction band necrosis.

These features can be recognized in cases where the perfusion was not restored; reperfused infarcts can have other hallmarks, such as contraction band necrosis.[83]

Prevention

The risk of a recurrent myocardial infarction decreases with strict blood pressure management and lifestyle changes, chiefly smoking cessation, regular exercise, a sensible diet for patients with heart disease, and limitation of alcohol intake.

Patients are usually commenced on several long-term medications post-MI, with the aim of preventing secondary cardiovascular events such as further myocardial infarctions, congestive heart failure or cerebrovascular accident (CVA). Unless contraindicated, such medications may include:[84] [85]

- Antiplatelet drug therapy such as aspirin and/or clopidogrel should be continued to reduce the risk of plaque rupture and recurrent myocardial infarction. Aspirin is first-line, owing to its low cost and comparable efficacy, with clopidogrel reserved for patients intolerant of aspirin. The combination of clopidogrel and aspirin may further reduce risk of cardiovascular events, however the risk of hemorrhage is increased.[86]
- Beta blocker therapy such as metoprolol or carvedilol should be commenced.[87] These have been particularly beneficial in high-risk patients such as those with left ventricular dysfunction and/or continuing cardiac ischaemia.[88] β-Blockers decrease mortality and morbidity. They also improve symptoms of cardiac ischemia in NSTEMI.

- ACE inhibitor therapy should be commenced 24–48 hours post-MI in hemodynamically-stable patients, particularly in patients with a history of MI, diabetes mellitus, hypertension, anterior location of infarct (as assessed by ECG), and/or evidence of left ventricular dysfunction. ACE inhibitors reduce mortality, the development of heart failure, and decrease ventricular remodelling post-MI.[89]
- Statin therapy has been shown to reduce mortality and morbidity post-MI.[90][91] The effects of statins may be more than their LDL lowering effects. The general consensus is that statins have plaque stabilization and multiple other ("pleiotropic") effects that may prevent myocardial infarction in addition to their effects on blood lipids.[92]
- The aldosterone antagonist agent eplerenone has been shown to further reduce risk of cardiovascular death post-MI in patients with heart failure and left ventricular dysfunction, when used in conjunction with standard therapies above.[93]
- Omega-3 fatty acids, commonly found in fish, have been shown to reduce mortality post-MI.[94] While the mechanism by which these fatty acids decrease mortality is unknown, it has been postulated that the survival benefit is due to electrical stabilization and the prevention of ventricular fibrillation.[95] However, further studies in a high-risk subset have not shown a clear-cut decrease in potentially fatal arrhythmias due to omega-3 fatty acids.[96][97]

Management

A heart attack is a medical emergency which demands both immediate attention and activation of the emergency medical services. The ultimate goal of the management in the acute phase of the disease is to salvage as much myocardium as possible and prevent further complications. As time passes, the risk of damage to the heart muscle increases; hence the phrase that in myocardial infarction, "time is muscle," and "time wasted is muscle lost".[98]

Oxygen, aspirin, glyceryl trinitrate (nitroglycerin) and analgesia are usually administered as soon as possible. In many areas, first responders are trained to administer these prior to arrival at the hospital. Morphine is classically used if nitroglycerin is not effective due to its ability to dilate blood vessels, which may aid in blood flow to the heart as well as relieve pain. Morphine may also cause hypotension (usually in the setting of hypovolemia), and should be avoided in the case of right ventricular infarction. Moreover, the CRUSADE trial demonstrated an increase in mortality with administering morphine in the setting of NSTEMI.[99] A 2009 review of high flow oxygen in myocardial infarction found increased mortality and infarct size, calling into question the recommendation about its routine use.[15]

Of the front line agents, aspirin and streptokinase have been shown to markedly reduce mortality.[100] Streptokinase activates plasminogen, which is fibrinolytic (see section on thrombolysis below).

Once the diagnosis of myocardial infarction is confirmed, other pharmacologic agents are often given. These include beta blockers,[101][102] anticoagulation (typically with heparin),[1] and possibly additional antiplatelet agents such as clopidogrel.[1]

Cocaine associated myocardial infarction should be managed in a manner similar to other patients with acute coronary syndrome except beta blockers should not be used and benzodiazepines should be administered early.[103]

The treatment itself may have complications. If attempts to restore the blood flow are initiated after a critical period of only a few hours, the result may be a reperfusion injury instead of amelioration.[104]

First aid

As myocardial infarction is a common medical emergency, the signs are often part of first aid courses. The emergency action principles also apply in the case of myocardial infarction.

When symptoms of myocardial infarction occur, people wait an average of three hours, instead of doing what is recommended: calling for help immediately.[105] [106] Acting immediately by calling the emergency services can save your life for two reasons. First and most importantly, the emergency services can immedialetely save your life from primary ventricular fibrillation which occurs unexpectedly in more than 10% of all infarction especially during the first hour of symptoms and second, immediate treatment of myocardial infarction can prevent sustained damage to the heart ("time is muscle").[98]

Certain positions allow the patient to rest in a position which minimizes breathing difficulties. A half-sitting position with knees bent is often recommended. Access to more oxygen can be given by opening the window and widening the collar for easier breathing.

Aspirin can be given quickly (if the patient is not allergic to aspirin); but taking aspirin before calling the emergency medical services may be associated with unwanted delay.[107] Aspirin has an antiplatelet effect which inhibits formation of further thrombi (blood clots) that clog arteries. Chewing is the preferred method of administration, so that the Aspirin can be absorbed quickly. Dissolved soluble preparations or sublingual administration can also be used. U.S. guidelines recommend a dose of 162–325 mg.[108] Australian guidelines recommend a dose of 150–300 mg.[84]

Glyceryl trinitrate (nitroglycerin) sublingually (under the tongue) can be given if available.

If an automated external defibrillator (AED) is available the rescuer should immediately bring the AED to the patient's side and be prepared to follow its instructions, especially should the victim lose consciousness.

If possible the rescuer should obtain basic information from the victim, in case the patient is unable to answer questions once emergency medical technicians arrive. The victim's name and any information regarding the nature of the victim's pain will be useful to health care providers. The exact time that these symptoms started may be critical for determining what interventions can be safely attempted once the victim reaches the medical center. Other useful pieces of information include what the patient was doing at the onset of symptoms, and anything else that might give clues to the pathology of the chest pain. It is also very important to relay any actions that have been taken, such as the number or dose of aspirin or nitroglycerin given, to the EMS personnel.

Other general first aid principles include monitoring pulse, breathing, level of consciousness and, if possible, the blood pressure of the patient. In case of cardiac arrest, cardiopulmonary resuscitation (CPR) can be administered.

Automatic external defibrillation (AED)

Since the publication of data showing that the availability of automated external defibrillators (AEDs) in public places may significantly increase chances of survival, many of these have been installed in public buildings, public transport facilities, and in non-ambulance emergency vehicles (e.g. police cars and fire engines). AEDs analyze the heart's rhythm and determine whether the rhythm is amenable to defibrillation ("shockable"), as in ventricular tachycardia and ventricular fibrillation.

Emergency services

Emergency Medical Services (EMS) Systems vary considerably in their ability to evaluate and treat patients with suspected acute myocardial infarction. Some provide as little as first aid and early defibrillation. Others employ highly trained paramedics with sophisticated technology and advanced protocols.[109] Early access to EMS is promoted by a 9-1-1 system currently available to 90% of the population in the United States.[109] Paramedic services are capable of providing oxygen, IV access, sublingual nitroglycerine, morphine, and aspirin. Some advanced paramedic systems can also perform 12-lead ECGs. If an STEMI is recognized the paramedic may be able to contact the local PCI hospital and alert the emergency room physician, and staff of the suspected AMI. Some Paramedic services are capable of providing thrombolytic therapy in the prehospital setting.[110] [111]

With primary PCI emerging as the preferred therapy for ST segment elevation myocardial infarction, EMS can play a key role in reducing door to balloon intervals (the time from presentation to a hospital ER to the restoration of coronary artery blood flow) by performing a 12 lead ECG in the field and using this information to triage the patient to the most appropriate medical facility.[112] [113] [114] [115] In addition, the 12 lead ECG can be transmitted to the receiving hospital, which enables time saving decisions to be made prior to the patient's arrival. This may include a "cardiac alert" or "STEMI alert" that calls in off duty personnel in areas where the cardiac cath lab is not staffed 24 hours a day.[116] Even in the absence of a formal alerting program, prehospital 12 lead ECGs are independently associated with reduced door to treatment intervals in the emergency department.[117]

Reperfusion

The concept of reperfusion has become so central to the modern treatment of acute myocardial infarction, that we are said to be in the reperfusion era.[118] [119] Patients who present with suspected acute myocardial infarction and ST segment elevation (STEMI) or new bundle branch block on the 12 lead ECG are presumed to have an occlusive thrombosis in an epicardial coronary artery. They are therefore candidates for immediate reperfusion, either with thrombolytic therapy, percutaneous coronary intervention (PCI) or when these therapies are unsuccessful, bypass surgery.

Individuals without ST segment elevation are presumed to be experiencing either unstable angina (UA) or non-ST segment elevation myocardial infarction (NSTEMI). They receive many of the same initial therapies and are often stabilized with antiplatelet drugs and anticoagulated. If their condition remains (hemodynamically) stable, they can be offered either late coronary angiography with subsequent restoration of blood flow (revascularization), or non-invasive stress testing to determine if there is significant ischemia that would benefit from revascularization. If hemodynamic instability develops in individuals with NSTEMIs, they may undergo urgent coronary angiography and subsequent revascularization. The use of thrombolytic agents is contraindicated in this patient subset, however.[120]

The basis for this distinction in treatment regimens is that ST segment elevations on an ECG are typically due to complete occlusion of a coronary artery. On the other hand, in NSTEMIs there is typically a sudden narrowing of a coronary artery with preserved (but diminished) flow to the distal myocardium. Anticoagulation and antiplatelet agents are given to prevent the narrowed artery from occluding.

At least 10% of patients with STEMI don't develop myocardial necrosis (as evidenced by a rise in cardiac markers) and subsequent Q waves on EKG after reperfusion therapy. Such a successful restoration of flow to the infarct-related artery during an acute myocardial infarction is known as "aborting" the myocardial infarction. If treated within the hour, about 25% of STEMIs can be aborted.[121]

Thrombolytic therapy

Thrombolytic therapy is indicated for the treatment of STEMI if the drug can be administered within 12 hours of the onset of symptoms, the patient is eligible based on exclusion criteria, and primary PCI is not immediately available.[1] The effectiveness of thrombolytic therapy is highest in the first 2 hours. After 12 hours, the risk associated with thrombolytic therapy outweighs any benefit.[120] [122] Because irreversible injury occurs within 2–4 hours of the infarction, there is a limited window of time available for reperfusion to work.

Thrombolytic drugs are contraindicated for the treatment of unstable angina and NSTEMI[120] [123] and for the treatment of individuals with evidence of cardiogenic shock.[124]

Although no perfect thrombolytic agent exists, an ideal thrombolytic drug would lead to rapid reperfusion, have a high sustained patency rate, be specific for recent thrombi, be easily and rapidly administered, create a low risk for intra-cerebral and systemic bleeding, have no antigenicity, adverse hemodynamic effects, or clinically significant drug interactions, and be cost effective.[125] Currently available thrombolytic agents include streptokinase, urokinase, and alteplase (recombinant tissue plasminogen activator, rtPA). More recently, thrombolytic agents similar in structure to rtPA such as reteplase and tenecteplase have been used. These newer agents boast efficacy at least as good as rtPA with significantly easier administration. The thrombolytic agent used in a particular individual is based on institution preference and the age of the patient.

Depending on the thrombolytic agent being used, adjuvant anticoagulation with heparin or low molecular weight heparin may be of benefit.[126] [127] With TPa and related agents (reteplase and tenecteplase), heparin is needed to maintain coronary artery patency. Because of the anticoagulant effect of fibrinogen depletion with streptokinase[128] and urokinase[129] [130] [131] treatment, it is less necessary there.[126]

Intracranial bleeding (ICB) and subsequent cerebrovascular accident (CVA) is a serious side effect of thrombolytic use. The risk of ICB is dependent on a number of factors, including a previous episode of intracranial bleed, age of the individual, and the thrombolytic regimen that is being used. In general, the risk of ICB due to thrombolytic use for the treatment of an acute myocardial infarction is between 0.5 and 1 percent.[126]

Thrombolytic therapy to abort a myocardial infarction is not always effective. The degree of effectiveness of a thrombolytic agent is dependent on the time since the myocardial infarction began, with the best results occurring if the thrombolytic agent is used within two hours of the onset of symptoms.[111] [132] If the individual presents more than 12 hours after symptoms commenced, the risk of intracranial bleed are considered higher than the benefits of the thrombolytic agent.[133] Failure rates of thrombolytics can be as high as 20% or higher.[134] In cases of failure of the thrombolytic agent to open the infarct-related coronary artery, the patient is then either treated conservatively with anticoagulants and allowed to "complete the infarction" or percutaneous coronary intervention (PCI, see below) is then performed. Percutaneous coronary intervention in this setting is known as "rescue PCI" or "salvage PCI". Complications, particularly bleeding, are significantly higher with rescue PCI than with primary PCI due to the action of the thrombolytic agent.

Percutaneous coronary intervention

The benefit of prompt, expertly performed primary percutaneous coronary intervention over thrombolytic therapy for acute ST elevation myocardial infarction is now well established.[135] [136] [137] When performed rapidly by an experienced team, primary PCI restores flow in the culprit artery in more than 95% of patients compared with the spontaneous recanalization rate of about 65%.[135] Logistic and economic obstacles seem to hinder a more widespread application of percutaneous coronary intervention (PCI) via cardiac catheterization,[138] although the feasibility of regionalized PCI for STEMI is currently being explored in the United States.[139] The use of percutaneous coronary intervention as a therapy to abort a myocardial infarction is known as primary PCI. The goal of primary PCI is to open

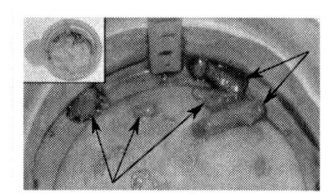

Thrombus material (in a cup, upper left corner) removed from a coronary artery during a percutaneous coronary intervention to abort a myocardial infarction. Five pieces of thrombus are shown (arrow heads).

the artery as soon as possible, and preferably within 90 minutes of the patient presenting to the emergency room. This time is referred to as the door-to-balloon time. Few hospitals can provide PCI within the 90 minute interval,[140] which prompted the American College of Cardiology (ACC) to launch a national Door to Balloon (D2B) Initiative in November 2006. Over 800 hospitals have joined the D2B Alliance as of March 16, 2007.[141]

One particularly successful implementation of a primary PCI protocol is in the Calgary Health Region under the auspices of the Libin Cardiovascular Institute of Alberta. Under this model, EMS teams responding to an emergency electronically transmit the ECG directly to a digital archiving system that allows emergency room physicians and/or cardiologists to immediately confirm the diagnosis. This in turn allows for redirection of the EMS teams to facilities prepped to conduct time-critical angioplasty, based on the ECG analysis. In an article published in the Canadian

Medical Association Journal in June 2007, the Calgary implementation resulted in a median time to treatment of 62 minutes.[142]

The current guidelines in the United States restrict primary PCI to hospitals with available emergency bypass surgery as a backup,[1] but this is not the case in other parts of the world.[143]

Primary PCI involves performing a coronary angiogram to determine the anatomical location of the infarcting vessel, followed by balloon angioplasty (and frequently deployment of an intracoronary stent) of the thrombosed arterial segment. In some settings, an extraction catheter may be used to attempt to aspirate (remove) the thrombus prior to balloon angioplasty. While the use of intracoronary stents do not improve the short term outcomes in primary PCI, the use of stents is widespread because of the decreased rates of procedures to treat restenosis compared to balloon angioplasty.[144]

Adjuvant therapy during primary PCI includes intravenous heparin, aspirin, and clopidogrel. Glycoprotein IIb/IIIa inhibitors are often used in the setting of primary PCI to reduce the risk of ischemic complications during the procedure.[145] [146] Due to the number of antiplatelet agents and anticoagulants used during primary PCI, the risk of bleeding associated with the procedure is higher than during an elective PCI.[147]

Coronary artery bypass surgery

Despite the guidelines, emergency bypass surgery for the treatment of an acute myocardial infarction (MI) is less common than PCI or medical management. In an analysis of patients in the U.S. National Registry of Myocardial Infarction (NRMI) from January 1995 to May 2004, the percentage of patients with cardiogenic shock treated with primary PCI rose from 27.4% to 54.4%, while the increase in CABG treatment was only from 2.1% to 3.2%.[148]

Emergency coronary artery bypass graft surgery (CABG) is usually undertaken to simultaneously treat a mechanical complication, such as a ruptured papillary muscle, or a ventricular septal defect, with ensuing cardiogenic shock.[149] In uncomplicated MI, the mortality rate can be high when the surgery is performed immediately following the infarction.[150] If this option is entertained, the patient should be stabilized prior to surgery, with supportive interventions such as the use of an intra-aortic balloon pump.[151] In patients developing cardiogenic shock after a myocardial infarction, both PCI and CABG are satisfactory treatment options, with similar survival rates.[152] [153]

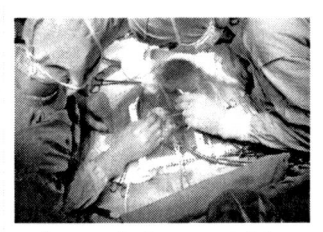

Coronary artery bypass surgery during mobilization (freeing) of the right coronary artery from its surrounding tissue, adipose tissue (yellow). The tube visible at the bottom is the aortic cannula (returns blood from the HLM). The tube above it (obscured by the surgeon on the right) is the venous cannula (receives blood from the body). The patient's heart is stopped and the aorta is cross-clamped. The patient's head (not seen) is at the bottom.

Coronary artery bypass surgery involves an artery or vein from the patient being implanted to bypass narrowings or occlusions on the coronary arteries. Several arteries and veins can be used, however internal mammary artery grafts have demonstrated significantly better long-term patency rates than great saphenous vein grafts.[154] In patients with two or more coronary arteries affected, bypass surgery is associated with higher long-term survival rates compared to percutaneous interventions.[155] In patients with single vessel disease, surgery is comparably safe and effective, and may be a treatment option in selected cases.[156] Bypass surgery has higher costs initially, but becomes cost-effective in the long term.[157] A surgical bypass graft is more invasive initially but bears less risk of recurrent procedures (but these may be again minimally invasive).[156]

Monitoring for arrhythmias

Additional objectives are to prevent life-threatening arrhythmias or conduction disturbances. This requires monitoring in a coronary care unit and protocolised administration of antiarrhythmic agents. Antiarrhythmic agents are typically only given to individuals with life-threatening arrhythmias after a myocardial infarction and not to suppress the ventricular ectopy that is often seen after a myocardial infarction.[158] [159] [160]

Austere environments

Wilderness first aid

In wilderness first aid, a possible heart attack justifies evacuation by the fastest available means, including MEDEVAC, even in the earliest or precursor stages. The patient will rapidly be incapable of further exertion and have to be carried out.

Air travel

Certified personnel traveling by commercial aircraft may be able to assist an MI patient by using the on-board first aid kit, which may contain some cardiac drugs (such as glyceryl trinitrate spray, aspirin, or opioid painkillers), an AED,[161] and oxygen. Pilots may divert the flight to land at a nearby airport. Cardiac monitors are being introduced by some airlines, and they can be used by both on-board and ground-based physicians.[162]

Rehabilitation

Cardiac rehabilitation aims to optimize function and quality of life in those afflicted with a heart disease. This can be with the help of a physician, or in the form of a cardiac rehabilitation program.[163]

Physical exercise is an important part of rehabilitation after a myocardial infarction, with beneficial effects on cholesterol levels, blood pressure, weight, stress and mood.[163] Some patients become afraid of exercising because it might trigger another infarct.[164] Patients are stimulated to exercise, and should only avoid certain exerting activities. Local authorities may place limitations on driving motorised vehicles.[165] Some people are afraid to have sex after a heart attack. Most people can resume sexual activities after 3 to 4 weeks. The amount of activity needs to be dosed to the patient's possibilities.[166]

New therapies under investigation

Patients who receive stem cell treatment by coronary artery injections of stem cells derived from their own bone marrow after a myocardial infarction (MI) show improvements in left ventricular ejection fraction and end-diastolic volume not seen with placebo. The larger the initial infarct size, the greater the effect of the infusion. Clinical trials of progenitor cell infusion as a treatment approach to ST elevation MI are proceeding.[167]

There are currently 3 biomaterial and tissue engineering approaches for the treatment of MI, but these are in an even earlier stage of medical research, so many questions and issues need to be addressed before they can be applied to patients. The first involves polymeric left ventricular restraints in the prevention of heart failure. The second utilizes *in vitro* engineered cardiac tissue, which is subsequently implanted *in vivo*. The final approach entails injecting cells and/or a scaffold into the myocardium to create *in situ* engineered cardiac tissue.[168]

Complications

Complications may occur immediately following the heart attack (in the acute phase), or may need time to develop (a chronic problem). After an infarction, an obvious complication is a second infarction, which may occur in the domain of another atherosclerotic coronary artery, or in the same zone if there are any live cells left in the infarct.

Congestive heart failure

A myocardial infarction may compromise the function of the heart as a pump for the circulation, a state called heart failure. There are different types of heart failure; left- or right-sided (or bilateral) heart failure may occur depending on the affected part of the heart, and it is a low-output type of failure. If one of the heart valves is affected, this may cause dysfunction, such as mitral regurgitation in the case of left-sided coronary occlusion that disrupts the blood supply of the papillary muscles. The incidence of heart failure is particularly high in patients with diabetes and requires special management strategies.[169]

Myocardial rupture

Myocardial rupture is most common three to five days after myocardial infarction, commonly of small degree, but may occur one day to three weeks later. In the modern era of early revascularization and intensive pharmacotherapy as treatment for MI, the incidence of myocardial rupture is about 1% of all MIs.[170] This may occur in the free walls of the ventricles, the septum between them, the papillary muscles, or less commonly the atria. Rupture occurs because of increased pressure against the weakened walls of the heart chambers due to heart muscle that cannot pump blood out effectively. The weakness may also lead to ventricular aneurysm, a localized dilation or ballooning of the heart chamber.

Risk factors for myocardial rupture include completion of infarction (no revascularization performed), female sex, advanced age, and a lack of a previous history of myocardial infarction.[170] In addition, the risk of rupture is higher in individuals who are revascularized with a thrombolytic agent than with PCI.[171] [172] The shear stress between the infarcted segment and the surrounding normal myocardium (which may be hypercontractile in the post-infarction period) makes it a nidus for rupture.[173]

Rupture is usually a catastrophic event that may result a life-threatening process known as cardiac tamponade, in which blood accumulates within the pericardium or heart sac, and compresses the heart to the point where it cannot pump effectively. Rupture of the intraventricular septum (the muscle separating the left and right ventricles) causes a ventricular septal defect with shunting of blood through the defect from the left side of the heart to the right side of the heart, which can lead to right ventricular failure as well as pulmonary overcirculation. Rupture of the papillary muscle may also lead to acute mitral regurgitation and subsequent pulmonary edema and possibly even cardiogenic shock.

Life-threatening arrhythmia

Since the electrical characteristics of the infarcted tissue change (see pathophysiology section), arrhythmias are a frequent complication.[174] The re-entry phenomenon may cause rapid heart rates (ventricular tachycardia and even ventricular fibrillation), and ischemia in the electrical conduction system of the heart may cause a complete heart block (when the impulse from the sinoatrial node, the normal cardiac pacemaker, does not reach the heart chambers).[175] [176]

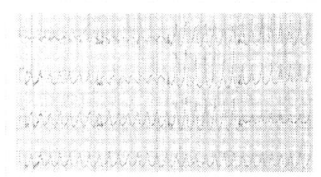

A 12 lead electrocardiogram showing ventricular tachycardia.

Pericarditis

As a reaction to the damage of the heart muscle, inflammatory cells are attracted. The inflammation may reach out and affect the heart sac. This is called pericarditis. In Dressler's syndrome, this occurs several weeks after the initial event.

Cardiogenic shock

A complication that may occur in the acute setting soon after a myocardial infarction or in the weeks following it is cardiogenic shock. Cardiogenic shock is defined as a hemodynamic state in which the heart cannot produce enough of a cardiac output to supply an adequate amount of oxygenated blood to the tissues of the body.

While the data on performing interventions on individuals with cardiogenic shock is sparse, trial data suggests a long-term mortality benefit in undergoing revascularization if the individual is less than 75 years old and if the onset of the acute myocardial infarction is less than 36 hours and the onset of cardiogenic shock is less than 18 hours.[124] If the patient with cardiogenic shock is not going to be revascularized, aggressive hemodynamic support is warranted, with insertion of an intra-aortic balloon pump if not contraindicated.[124] If diagnostic coronary angiography does not reveal a culprit blockage that is the cause of the cardiogenic shock, the prognosis is poor.[124]

Prognosis

The prognosis for patients with myocardial infarction varies greatly, depending on the patient, the condition itself and the given treatment. Using simple variables which are immediately available in the emergency room, patients with a higher risk of adverse outcome can be identified. For example, one study found that 0.4% of patients with a low risk profile had died after 90 days, whereas the mortality rate in high risk patients was 21.1%.[177]

For the period 2005 - 2008 in the United States the median mortality at 30 days was 16.6% with a range from 10.9% to 24.9% depending on the hospital which one looks at.[178]

Although studies differ in the identified variables, some of the more reproduced risk stratifiers include age, hemodynamic parameters (such as heart failure, cardiac arrest on admission, systolic blood pressure, or Killip class of two or greater), ST-segment deviation, diabetes, serum creatinine concentration, peripheral vascular disease and elevation of cardiac markers.[177] [179] [180]

Assessment of left ventricular ejection fraction may increase the predictive power of some risk stratification models.[181] The prognostic importance of Q-waves is debated.[182] Prognosis is significantly worsened if a mechanical complication (papillary muscle rupture, myocardial free wall rupture, and so on) were to occur.[171]

There is evidence that case fatality of myocardial infarction has been improving over the years in all ethnicities.[183]

Epidemiology

Myocardial infarction is a common presentation of ischemic heart disease. The WHO estimated that in 2002, 12.6 percent of deaths worldwide were from ischemic heart disease.[1] Ischemic heart disease is the leading cause of death in developed countries, but third to AIDS and lower respiratory infections in developing countries.[184]

In the United States, diseases of the heart are the leading cause of death, causing a higher mortality than cancer (malignant neoplasms).[185] Coronary heart disease is responsible for 1 in 5 deaths in the U.S..This means that roughly every 65 seconds, an American dies of a coronary event.

In India, cardiovascular disease (CVD) is the leading cause of death.[186] The deaths due to CVD in India were 32% of all deaths in 2007 and are expected to rise from 1.17 million in 1990 and 1.59 million in 2000 to 2.03 million in 2010.[187] Although a relatively new epidemic in India, it has quickly become a major health issue with deaths due to CVD expected to double during 1985-2015.[188] [189] Mortality estimates due to CVD vary widely by state, ranging from 10% in Meghalaya to 49% in Punjab (percentage of all deaths). Punjab (49%), Goa (42%), Tamil Nadu (36%)

and Andhra Pradesh (31%) have the highest CVD related mortality estimates.[190] State-wise differences are correlated with prevalence of specific dietary risk factors in the states. Moderate physical exercise is associated with reduced incidence of CVD in India (those who exercise have less than half the risk of those who don't).[188] CVD also affects Native Americans at a younger age (in their 30s and 40s) than is typical in other countries.

Legal implications

At common law, a myocardial infarction is generally a disease, but may sometimes be an injury. This has implications for no-fault insurance schemes such as workers' compensation. A heart attack is generally not covered;[191] however, it may be a work-related injury if it results, for example, from unusual emotional stress or unusual exertion.[192] Additionally, in some jurisdictions, heart attacks suffered by persons in particular occupations such as police officers may be classified as line-of-duty injuries by statute or policy. In some countries or states, a person who has suffered from a myocardial infarction may be prevented from participating in activity that puts other people's lives at risk, for example driving a car or flying an airplane.[165]

External links

- American Heart Association's Heart Attack web site [193] - Information and resources for preventing, recognizing and treating heart attack.
- Heartscore: an interactive tool for prediction and risk management of stroke and heart attack [55] (EU)
- Heart Attack [194] - overview of resources from MedlinePlus.
- Risk Assessment Tool for Estimating 10-year Risk of Having a Heart Attack [195] - based on information of the Framingham Heart Study, from the United States National Heart, Lung and Blood Institute

References

[1] http://apps.who.int/classifications/apps/icd/icd10online/?gi20.htm+i21
[2] http://apps.who.int/classifications/apps/icd/icd10online/?gi20.htm+i22
[3] http://www.icd9data.com/getICD9Code.ashx?icd9=410
[4] http://www.diseasesdatabase.com/ddb8664.htm
[5] http://www.nlm.nih.gov/medlineplus/ency/article/000195.htm
[6] http://www.emedicine.com/med/topic1567.htm
[7] http://www.emedicine.com/emerg/topic327.htm#
[8] http://www.emedicine.com/ped/topic2520.htm#
[9] http://www.nlm.nih.gov/cgi/mesh/2009/MB_cgi?field=uid&term=D009203
[10] Kosuge, M; Kimura K, Ishikawa T et al. (March 2006). "Differences between men and women in terms of clinical features of ST-segment elevation acute myocardial infarction" (http://www.jstage.jst.go.jp/article/circj/70/3/222/_pdf). *Circulation Journal* **70** (3): 222–226. doi: 10.1253/circj.70.222 (http://dx.doi.org/10.1253/circj.70.222). PMID 16501283 (http://www.ncbi.nlm.nih.gov/pubmed/16501283). . Retrieved 2008-05-31.
[11] Robert Beaglehole, *et al.* (2004) (PDF). *The World Health Report 2004 - Changing History* (http://www.who.int/entity/whr/2004/en/report04_en.pdf). World Health Organization. pp. 120–4. ISBN 92-4-156265-X. .
[12] Bax L, Algra A, Mali WP, Edlinger M, Beutler JJ, van der Graaf Y (2008). "Renal function as a risk indicator for cardiovascular events in 3216 patients with manifest arterial disease" (http://linkinghub.elsevier.com/retrieve/pii/S0021-9150(07)00768-X). *Atherosclerosis* **200** (1): 184. doi: 10.1016/j.atherosclerosis.2007.12.006 (http://dx.doi.org/10.1016/j.atherosclerosis.2007.12.006). PMID 18241872 (http://www.ncbi.nlm.nih.gov/pubmed/18241872). .
[13] Pearte CA, Furberg CD, O'Meara ES, *et al.* (2006). "Characteristics and baseline clinical predictors of future fatal versus nonfatal coronary heart disease events in older adults: the Cardiovascular Health Study" (http://circ.ahajournals.org/cgi/content/full/113/18/2177). *Circulation* **113** (18): 2177–85. doi: 10.1161/CIRCULATIONAHA.105.610352 (http://dx.doi.org/10.1161/CIRCULATIONAHA.105.610352). PMID 16651468 (http://www.ncbi.nlm.nih.gov/pubmed/16651468). .
[14] Erhardt L, Herlitz J, Bossaert L, *et al.* (2002). "Task force on the management of chest pain" (http://eurheartj.oxfordjournals.org/cgi/reprint/23/15/1153) (PDF). *Eur. Heart J.* **23** (15): 1153–76. doi: 10.1053/euhj.2002.3194 (http://dx.doi.org/10.1053/euhj.2002.3194). PMID 12206127 (http://www.ncbi.nlm.nih.gov/pubmed/12206127). .
[15] "Routine use of oxygen in the treatment of myocardial infarction: systematic review -- Wijesinghe et al. 95 (3): 198 -- Heart" (http://heart.bmj.com/cgi/content/full/95/3/198). .

[16] National Heart, Lung and Blood Institute. Heart Attack Warning Signs (http://www.nhlbi.nih.gov/actintime/haws/haws.htm). Retrieved November 22, 2006.
[17] Marcus GM, Cohen J, Varosy PD, et al. (2007). "The utility of gestures in patients with chest discomfort" (http://linkinghub.elsevier.com/retrieve/pii/S0002-9343(06)00668-1). Am. J. Med. 120 (1): 83–9. doi: 10.1016/j.amjmed.2006.05.045 (http://dx.doi.org/10.1016/j.amjmed.2006.05.045). PMID 17208083 (http://www.ncbi.nlm.nih.gov/pubmed/17208083). .
[18] Little RA, Frayn KN, Randall PE, et al. (1986). "Plasma catecholamines in the acute phase of the response to myocardial infarction" (http://www.pubmedcentral.nih.gov/articlerender.fcgi?tool=pmcentrez&artid=1285314). Arch Emerg Med 3 (1): 20–7. PMID 3524599 (http://www.ncbi.nlm.nih.gov/pubmed/3524599).
[19] Canto JG, Goldberg RJ, Hand MM, et al. (December 2007). "Symptom presentation of women with acute coronary syndromes: myth vs reality" (http://archinte.ama-assn.org/cgi/pmidlookup?view=long&pmid=18071161). Arch. Intern. Med. 167 (22): 2405–13. doi: 10.1001/archinte.167.22.2405 (http://dx.doi.org/10.1001/archinte.167.22.2405). PMID 18071161 (http://www.ncbi.nlm.nih.gov/pubmed/18071161). .
[20] McSweeney JC, Cody M, O'Sullivan P, Elberson K, Moser DK, Garvin BJ (2003). "Women's early warning symptoms of acute myocardial infarction". Circulation 108 (21): 2619–23. doi: 10.1161/01.CIR.0000097116.29625.7C (http://dx.doi.org/10.1161/01.CIR.0000097116.29625.7C). PMID 14597589 (http://www.ncbi.nlm.nih.gov/pubmed/14597589).
[21] D Lee, D Kulick, J Marks. Heart Attack (Myocardial Infarction) (http://www.medicinenet.com/heart_attack/article.htm) by MedicineNet.com . Retrieved November 28, 2006.
[22] Kannel WB. (1986). "Silent myocardial ischemia and infarction: insights from the Framingham Study". Cardiol Clin 4 (4): 583–91. PMID 3779719 (http://www.ncbi.nlm.nih.gov/pubmed/3779719).
[23] Davis TM, Fortun P, Mulder J, Davis WA, Bruce DG (2004). "Silent myocardial infarction and its prognosis in a community-based cohort of Type 2 diabetic patients: the Fremantle Diabetes Study". Diabetologia 47 (3): 395–9. doi: 10.1007/s00125-004-1344-4 (http://dx.doi.org/10.1007/s00125-004-1344-4). PMID 14963648 (http://www.ncbi.nlm.nih.gov/pubmed/14963648).
[24] *Rubin's Pathology - Clinicopathological Foundations of Medicine*. Maryland: Lippincott Williams & Wilkins. 2001. pp. 549. ISBN 0-7817-4733-3.
[25] Acute Coronary Syndrome (http://www.americanheart.org/presenter.jhtml?identifier=3010002). American Heart Association. Retrieved November 25, 2006.
[26] Boie ET (2005). "Initial evaluation of chest pain" (http://linkinghub.elsevier.com/retrieve/pii/S0733-8627(05)00059-3). Emerg. Med. Clin. North Am. 23 (4): 937–57. doi: 10.1016/j.emc.2005.07.007 (http://dx.doi.org/10.1016/j.emc.2005.07.007). PMID 16199332 (http://www.ncbi.nlm.nih.gov/pubmed/16199332). .
[27] Wilson PW, D'Agostino RB, Levy D, Belanger AM, Silbershatz H, Kannel WB. " Prediction of coronary heart disease using risk factor categories (http://circ.ahajournals.org/cgi/content/full/97/18/1837)". Circulation 1998; 97(18): 1837-47. PMID 9603539
[28] Saikku P, Leinonen M, Tenkanen L, Linnanmaki E, Ekman MR, Manninen V, Manttari M, Frick MH, Huttunen JK. (1992). "Chronic Chlamydia pneumoniae infection as a risk factor for coronary heart disease in the Helsinki Heart Study". Ann Intern Med 116 (4): 273–8. PMID 1733381 (http://www.ncbi.nlm.nih.gov/pubmed/1733381).
[29] Andraws R, Berger JS, Brown DL. (2005). "Effects of antibiotic therapy on outcomes of patients with coronary artery disease: a meta-analysis of randomized controlled trials". JAMA 293 (21): 2641–7. doi: 10.1001/jama.293.21.2641 (http://dx.doi.org/10.1001/jama.293.21.2641). PMID 15928286 (http://www.ncbi.nlm.nih.gov/pubmed/15928286).
[30] Muller JE, Stone PH, Turi ZG, et al. (1985). "Circadian variation in the frequency of onset of acute myocardial infarction". N. Engl. J. Med. 313 (21): 1315–22. PMID 2865677 (http://www.ncbi.nlm.nih.gov/pubmed/2865677).
[31] Beamer AD, Lee TH, Cook EF, et al. (1987). "Diagnostic implications for myocardial ischemia of the circadian variation of the onset of chest pain". Am. J. Cardiol. 60 (13): 998–1002. doi: 10.1016/0002-9149(87)90340-7 (http://dx.doi.org/10.1016/0002-9149(87)90340-7). PMID 3673917 (http://www.ncbi.nlm.nih.gov/pubmed/3673917).
[32] Cannon CP, McCabe CH, Stone PH, et al. (1997). "Circadian variation in the onset of unstable angina and non-Q-wave acute myocardial infarction (the TIMI III Registry and TIMI IIIB)" (http://linkinghub.elsevier.com/retrieve/pii/S0002914997007431). Am. J. Cardiol. 79 (3): 253–8. doi: 10.1016/S0002-9149(97)00743-1 (http://dx.doi.org/10.1016/S0002-9149(97)00743-1). PMID 9036740 (http://www.ncbi.nlm.nih.gov/pubmed/9036740). .
[33] Tofler GH, Brezinski D, Schafer AI, et al. (1987). "Concurrent morning increase in platelet aggregability and the risk of myocardial infarction and sudden cardiac death". N. Engl. J. Med. 316 (24): 1514–8. PMID 3587281 (http://www.ncbi.nlm.nih.gov/pubmed/3587281).
[34] Fantidis P, Perez De Prada T, Fernandez-Ortiz A, et al. (2002). "Morning cortisol production in coronary heart disease patients" (http://www.blackwell-synergy.com/openurl?genre=article&sid=nlm:pubmed&issn=0014-2972&date=2002&volume=32&issue=5&spage=304). Eur. J. Clin. Invest. 32 (5): 304–8. doi: 10.1046/j.1365-2362.2002.00988.x (http://dx.doi.org/10.1046/j.1365-2362.2002.00988.x). PMID 12027868 (http://www.ncbi.nlm.nih.gov/pubmed/12027868). .
[35] Yusuf S, Hawken S, Ounpuu S, Bautista L, Franzosi MG, Commerford P, Lang CC, Rumboldt Z, Onen CL, Lisheng L, Tanomsup S, Wangai P Jr, Razak F, Sharma AM, Anand SS; INTERHEART Study Investigators. (2005). "Obesity and the risk of myocardial infarction in 27,000 participants from 52 countries: a case-control study". Lancet 366 (9497): 1640–9. doi: 10.1016/S0140-6736(05)67663-5 (http://dx.doi.org/10.1016/S0140-6736(05)67663-5). PMID 16271645 (http://www.ncbi.nlm.nih.gov/pubmed/16271645).
[36] Jensen G, Nyboe J, Appleyard M, Schnohr P. (1991). "Risk factors for acute myocardial infarction in Copenhagen, II: Smoking, alcohol intake, physical activity, obesity, oral contraception, diabetes, lipids, and blood pressure". Eur Heart J 12 (3): 298–308. PMID 2040311 (http:/

/www.ncbi.nlm.nih.gov/pubmed/2040311).
[37] Nyboe J, Jensen G, Appleyard M, Schnohr P. (1989). "Risk factors for acute myocardial infarction in Copenhagen. I: Hereditary, educational and socioeconomic factors. Copenhagen City Heart Study". *Eur Heart J* **10** (10): 910–6. PMID 2598948 (http://www.ncbi.nlm.nih.gov/pubmed/2598948).
[38] Khader YS, Rice J, John L, Abueita O. (2003). "Oral contraceptives use and the risk of myocardial infarction: a meta-analysis". *Contraception* **68** (1): 11–7. doi: 10.1016/S0010-7824(03)00073-8 (http://dx.doi.org/10.1016/S0010-7824(03)00073-8). PMID 12878281 (http://www.ncbi.nlm.nih.gov/pubmed/12878281).
[39] Wilson AM, Ryan MC, Boyle AJ. (2006). "The novel role of C-reactive protein in cardiovascular disease: risk marker or pathogen". *Int J Cardiol* **106** (3): 291–7. doi: 10.1016/j.ijcard.2005.01.068 (http://dx.doi.org/10.1016/j.ijcard.2005.01.068). PMID 16337036 (http://www.ncbi.nlm.nih.gov/pubmed/16337036).
[40] Pearson TA, Mensah GA, Alexander RW, Anderson JL, Cannon RO 3rd, Criqui M, Fadl YY, Fortmann SP, Hong Y, Myers GL, Rifai N, Smith SC Jr, Taubert K, Tracy RP, Vinicor F; Centers for Disease Control and Prevention; American Heart Association. (2003). "Markers of inflammation and cardiovascular disease: application to clinical and public health practice: A statement for healthcare professionals from the Centers for Disease Control and Prevention and the American Heart Association" (http://circ.ahajournals.org/cgi/reprint/107/3/499.pdf) (PDF). *Circulation* **107** (3): 499–511. doi: 10.1161/01.CIR.0000052939.59093.45 (http://dx.doi.org/10.1161/01.CIR.0000052939.59093.45). PMID 12551878 (http://www.ncbi.nlm.nih.gov/pubmed/12551878). .
[41] Janket SJ, Baird AE, Chuang SK, Jones JA. (2003). "Meta-analysis of periodontal disease and risk of coronary heart disease and stroke". *Oral Surg Oral Med Oral Pathol Oral Radiol Endod.* **95** (5): 559–69. doi: 10.1038/sj.ebd.6400272 (http://dx.doi.org/10.1038/sj.ebd.6400272). PMID 12738947 (http://www.ncbi.nlm.nih.gov/pubmed/12738947).
[42] Pihlstrom BL, Michalowicz BS, Johnson NW. (2005). "Periodontal diseases". *Lancet* **366** (9499): 1809–20. doi: 10.1016/S0140-6736(05)67728-8 (http://dx.doi.org/10.1016/S0140-6736(05)67728-8). PMID 16298220 (http://www.ncbi.nlm.nih.gov/pubmed/16298220).
[43] Scannapieco FA, Bush RB, Paju S. (2003). "Associations between periodontal disease and risk for atherosclerosis, cardiovascular disease, and stroke. A systematic review". *Ann Periodontol* **8** (1): 38–53. doi: 10.1902/annals.2003.8.1.38 (http://dx.doi.org/10.1902/annals.2003.8.1.38). PMID 14971247 (http://www.ncbi.nlm.nih.gov/pubmed/14971247).
[44] D'Aiuto F, Parkar M, Nibali L, Suvan J, Lessem J, Tonetti MS. (2006). "Periodontal infections cause changes in traditional and novel cardiovascular risk factors: results from a randomized controlled clinical trial". *Am Heart J* **151** (5): 977–84. doi: 10.1016/j.ahj.2005.06.018 (http://dx.doi.org/10.1016/j.ahj.2005.06.018). PMID 16644317 (http://www.ncbi.nlm.nih.gov/pubmed/16644317).
[45] Lourbakos A, Yuan YP, Jenkins AL, Travis J, Andrade-Gordon P, Santulli R, Potempa J, Pike RN. (2001). "Activation of protease-activated receptors by gingipains from Porphyromonas gingivalis leads to platelet aggregation: a new trait in microbial pathogenicity" (http://bloodjournal.hematologylibrary.org/cgi/reprint/97/12/3790.pdf) (PDF). *Blood* **97** (12): 3790–7. doi: 10.1182/blood.V97.12.3790 (http://dx.doi.org/10.1182/blood.V97.12.3790). PMID 11389018 (http://www.ncbi.nlm.nih.gov/pubmed/11389018). .
[46] Qi M, Miyakawa H, Kuramitsu HK. (2003). "Porphyromonas gingivalis induces murine macrophage foam cell formation". *Microb Pathog* **35** (6): 259–67. doi: 10.1016/j.micpath.2003.07.002 (http://dx.doi.org/10.1016/j.micpath.2003.07.002). PMID 14580389 (http://www.ncbi.nlm.nih.gov/pubmed/14580389).
[47] Spahr A, Klein E, Khuseyinova N, Boeckh C, Muche R, Kunze M, Rothenbacher D, Pezeshki G, Hoffmeister A, Koenig W. (2006). "Periodontal infections and coronary heart disease: role of periodontal bacteria and importance of total pathogen burden in the Coronary Event and Periodontal Disease (CORODONT) study". *Arch Intern Med* **166** (5): 554–9. doi: 10.1001/archinte.166.5.554 (http://dx.doi.org/10.1001/archinte.166.5.554). PMID 16534043 (http://www.ncbi.nlm.nih.gov/pubmed/16534043).
[48] Warren-Gash C, Smeeth L, Hayward AC (2009). "Influenza as a trigger for acute myocardial infarction or death from cardiovascular disease: a systematic review". *Lancet Infect Dis* **9** (10): 601–610. doi: 10.1016/S1473-3099(09)70233-6 (http://dx.doi.org/10.1016/S1473-3099(09)70233-6).
[49] Davis TM, Balme M, Jackson D, Stuccio G, Bruce DG (October 2000). "The diagonal ear lobe crease (Frank's sign) is not associated with coronary artery disease or retinopathy in type 2 diabetes: the Fremantle Diabetes Study". *Aust N Z J Med* **30** (5): 573–7. PMID 11108067 (http://www.ncbi.nlm.nih.gov/pubmed/11108067).
[50] Lichstein E, Chadda KD, Naik D, Gupta PK. (1974). "Diagonal ear-lobe crease: prevalence and implications as a coronary risk factor". *N Engl J Med* **290** (11): 615–6. PMID 4812503 (http://www.ncbi.nlm.nih.gov/pubmed/4812503).
[51] Miric D, Fabijanic D, Giunio L, Eterovic D, Culic V, Bozic I, Hozo I. (1998). "Dermatological indicators of coronary risk: a case-control study". *Int J Cardiol* **67** (3): 251–5. doi: 10.1016/S0167-5273(98)00313-1 (http://dx.doi.org/10.1016/S0167-5273(98)00313-1). PMID 9894707 (http://www.ncbi.nlm.nih.gov/pubmed/9894707).
[52] Greenland P, LaBree L, Azen SP, Doherty TM, Detrano RC (2004). "Coronary artery calcium score combined with Framingham score for risk prediction in asymptomatic individuals" (http://jama.ama-assn.org/cgi/pmidlookup?view=long&pmid=14722147). *JAMA* **291** (2): 210–5. doi: 10.1001/jama.291.2.210 (http://dx.doi.org/10.1001/jama.291.2.210). PMID 14722147 (http://www.ncbi.nlm.nih.gov/pubmed/14722147). .
[53] Detrano R, Guerci AD, Carr JJ, et al. (2008). "Coronary calcium as a predictor of coronary events in four racial or ethnic groups" (http://content.nejm.org/cgi/pmidlookup?view=short&pmid=18367736&promo=ONFLNS19). *N. Engl. J. Med.* **358** (13): 1336–45. doi: 10.1056/NEJMoa072100 (http://dx.doi.org/10.1056/NEJMoa072100). PMID 18367736 (http://www.ncbi.nlm.nih.gov/pubmed/18367736). .

[54] Arad Y, Goodman KJ, Roth M, Newstein D, Guerci AD (2005). "Coronary calcification, coronary disease risk factors, C-reactive protein, and atherosclerotic cardiovascular disease events: the St. Francis Heart Study" (http://linkinghub.elsevier.com/retrieve/pii/S0735-1097(05)01031-4). *J. Am. Coll. Cardiol.* **46** (1): 158–65. doi: 10.1016/j.jacc.2005.02.088 (http://dx.doi.org/10.1016/j.jacc.2005.02.088). PMID 15992651 (http://www.ncbi.nlm.nih.gov/pubmed/15992651). .
[55] http://www.heartscore.org
[56] Krijnen PA, Nijmeijer R, Meijer CJ, Visser CA, Hack CE, Niessen HW. (2002). "Apoptosis in myocardial ischaemia and infarction" (http://www.pubmedcentral.nih.gov/articlerender.fcgi?tool=pmcentrez&artid=1769793). *J Clin Pathol* **55** (11): 801–11. doi: 10.1136/jcp.55.11.801 (http://dx.doi.org/10.1136/jcp.55.11.801). PMID 12401816 (http://www.ncbi.nlm.nih.gov/pubmed/12401816).
[57] Myocardial infarction: diagnosis and investigations (http://www.gpnotebook.co.uk/simplepage.cfm?ID=892665874&linkID=23278&cook=yes) - GPnotebook, retrieved November 27, 2006.
[58] DE Fenton et al. Myocardial infarction (http://www.emedicine.com/EMERG/topic327.htm#section~workup) - eMedicine, retrieved November 27, 2006.
[59] HEART SCAN (http://www.ucl.ac.uk/nuclear-medicine/Patient_Information/Scans/Cardiac.htm) - Patient information from University College London. Retrieved November 27, 2006.
[60] Skoufis E, McGhie AI (1998). "Radionuclide techniques for the assessment of myocardial viability" (http://www.pubmedcentral.nih.gov/articlerender.fcgi?tool=pmcentrez&artid=325572). *Tex Heart Inst J* **25** (4): 272–9. PMID 9885104 (http://www.ncbi.nlm.nih.gov/pubmed/9885104).
[61] Anonymous (March 1979). "Nomenclature and criteria for diagnosis of ischemic heart disease. Report of the Joint International Society and Federation of Cardiology/World Health Organization task force on standardization of clinical nomenclature". *Circulation* **59** (3): 607–9. PMID 761341 (http://www.ncbi.nlm.nih.gov/pubmed/761341).
[62] Alpert JS, Thygesen K, Antman E, Bassand JP. (2000). "Myocardial infarction redefined--a consensus document of The Joint European Society of Cardiology/American College of Cardiology Committee for the redefinition of myocardial infarction". *J Am Coll Cardiol* **36** (3): 959–69. doi: 10.1016/S0735-1097(00)00804-4 (http://dx.doi.org/10.1016/S0735-1097(00)00804-4). PMID 10987628 (http://www.ncbi.nlm.nih.gov/pubmed/10987628).
[63] S. Garas et al.. Myocardial Infarction (http://www.emedicine.com/med/topic1567.htm). eMedicine. Retrieved November 22, 2006.
[64] Kasper DL, Braunwald E, Fauci AS, Hauser SL, Longo DL, Jameson JL. *Harrison's Principles of Internal Medicine*. p. 1444. New York: McGraw-Hill, 2005. ISBN 0-07-139140-1.
[65] Cannon CP at al. *Management of Acute Coronary Syndromes*. p. 175. New Jersey: Humana Press, 1999. ISBN 0-89603-552-2.
[66] Selker HP, Zalenski RJ, Antman EM, et al. (January 1997). "An evaluation of technologies for identifying acute cardiac ischemia in the emergency department: executive summary of a National Heart Attack Alert Program Working Group Report". *Ann Emerg Med* **29** (1): 1–12. doi: 10.1016/S0196-0644(97)70297-X (http://dx.doi.org/10.1016/S0196-0644(97)70297-X). PMID 8998085 (http://www.ncbi.nlm.nih.gov/pubmed/8998085).
[67] Masoudi FA, Magid DJ, Vinson DR, et al. (October 2006). "Implications of the failure to identify high-risk electrocardiogram findings for the quality of care of patients with acute myocardial infarction: results of the Emergency Department Quality in Myocardial Infarction (EDQMI) study" (http://circ.ahajournals.org/cgi/content/full/114/15/1565). *Circulation* **114** (15): 1565–71. doi: 10.1161/CIRCULATIONAHA.106.623652 (http://dx.doi.org/10.1161/CIRCULATIONAHA.106.623652). PMID 17015790 (http://www.ncbi.nlm.nih.gov/pubmed/17015790). .
[68] "2005 American Heart Association Guidelines for Cardiopulmonary Resuscitation and Emergency Cardiovascular Care - Part 8: Stabilization of the Patient With Acute Coronary Syndromes" (http://circ.ahajournals.org/cgi/content/full/112/24_suppl/IV-89). *Circulation* **112**: IV–89–IV–110. 2005. doi: 10.1161/CIRCULATIONAHA.105.166561 (http://dx.doi.org/10.1161/CIRCULATIONAHA.105.166561). .
[69] Somers MP, Brady WJ, Perron AD, Mattu A (May 2002). "The prominant [sic] T wave: electrocardiographic differential diagnosis". *Am J Emerg Med* **20** (3): 243–51. doi: 10.1053/ajem.2002.32630 (http://dx.doi.org/10.1053/ajem.2002.32630). PMID 11992348 (http://www.ncbi.nlm.nih.gov/pubmed/11992348).
[70] Smith SW, Whitwam W (February 2006). "Acute coronary syndromes". *Emerg. Med. Clin. North Am.* **24** (1): 53–89, vi. doi: 10.1016/j.emc.2005.08.008 (http://dx.doi.org/10.1016/j.emc.2005.08.008). PMID 16308113 (http://www.ncbi.nlm.nih.gov/pubmed/16308113).
[71] Van Mieghem C, Sabbe M, Knockaert D (April 2004). "The clinical value of the ECG in noncardiac conditions" (http://www.chestjournal.org/cgi/content/full/125/4/1561). *Chest* **125** (4): 1561–76. doi: 10.1378/chest.125.4.1561 (http://dx.doi.org/10.1378/chest.125.4.1561). PMID 15078775 (http://www.ncbi.nlm.nih.gov/pubmed/15078775). .
[72] Brady WJ, Perron AD, Martin ML, Beagle C, Aufderheide TP (January 2001). "Cause of ST segment abnormality in ED chest pain patients". *Am J Emerg Med* **19** (1): 25–8. doi: 10.1053/ajem.2001.18029 (http://dx.doi.org/10.1053/ajem.2001.18029). PMID 11146012 (http://www.ncbi.nlm.nih.gov/pubmed/11146012).
[73] Wang K, Asinger RW, Marriott HJ (November 2003). "ST-segment elevation in conditions other than acute myocardial infarction". *N. Engl. J. Med.* **349** (22): 2128–35. doi: 10.1056/NEJMra022580 (http://dx.doi.org/10.1056/NEJMra022580). PMID 14645641 (http://www.ncbi.nlm.nih.gov/pubmed/14645641).
[74] Brady WJ, Chan TC, Pollack M (January 2000). "Electrocardiographic manifestations: patterns that confound the EKG diagnosis of acute myocardial infarction-left bundle branch block, ventricular paced rhythm, and left ventricular hypertrophy" (http://linkinghub.elsevier.com/

retrieve/pii/S0736-4679(99)00178-X). *J Emerg Med* **18** (1): 71–8. doi: 10.1016/S0736-4679(99)00178-X (http://dx.doi.org/10.1016/S0736-4679(99)00178-X). PMID 10645842 (http://www.ncbi.nlm.nih.gov/pubmed/10645842). .

[75] Brady WJ, Perron AD, Chan T (April 2001). "Electrocardiographic ST-segment elevation: correct identification of acute myocardial infarction (AMI) and non-AMI syndromes by emergency physicians". *Acad Emerg Med* **8** (4): 349–60. doi: 10.1111/j.1553-2712.2001.tb02113.x (http://dx.doi.org/10.1111/j.1553-2712.2001.tb02113.x). PMID 11282670 (http://www.ncbi.nlm.nih.gov/pubmed/11282670).

[76] Eisenman A (2006). "Troponin assays for the diagnosis of myocardial infarction and acute coronary syndrome: where do we stand?". *Expert Rev Cardiovasc Ther* **4** (4): 509–14. doi: 10.1586/14779072.4.4.509 (http://dx.doi.org/10.1586/14779072.4.4.509). PMID 16918269 (http://www.ncbi.nlm.nih.gov/pubmed/16918269).

[77] Aviles RJ, Askari AT, Lindahl B, Wallentin L, Jia G, Ohman EM, Mahaffey KW, Newby LK, Califf RM, Simoons ML, Topol EJ, Berger P, Lauer MS (2002). "Troponin T levels in patients with acute coronary syndromes, with or without renal dysfunction". *N Engl J Med* **346** (26): 2047–52. doi: 10.1056/NEJMoa013456 (http://dx.doi.org/10.1056/NEJMoa013456). PMID 12087140 (http://www.ncbi.nlm.nih.gov/pubmed/12087140). . Summary for laymen (http://www.cmaj.ca/cgi/content/full/167/6/671)

[78] Apple FS, Wu AH, Mair J, *et al.* (2005). "Future biomarkers for detection of ischemia and risk stratification in acute coronary syndrome" (http://www.clinchem.org/cgi/content/full/51/5/810). *Clin. Chem.* **51** (5): 810–24. doi: 10.1373/clinchem.2004.046292 (http://dx.doi.org/10.1373/clinchem.2004.046292). PMID 15774573 (http://www.ncbi.nlm.nih.gov/pubmed/15774573). .

[79] Braunwald E, Antman EM, Beasley JW, Califf RM, Cheitlin MD, Hochman JS, Jones RH, Kereiakes D, Kupersmith J, Levin TN, Pepine CJ, Schaeffer JW, Smith EE III, Steward DE, Théroux P. (2002). "ACC/AHA 2002 guideline update for the management of patients with unstable angina and non–ST-segment elevation myocardial infarction: a report of the American College of Cardiology/American Heart Association Task Force on Practice Guidelines (Committee on the Management of Patients With Unstable Angina)" (http://www.acc.org/qualityandscience/clinical/guidelines/unstable/incorporated/UA_incorporated.pdf) (PDF). *J Am Coll Cardiol* **40** (7): 1366–74. PMID 12383588 (http://www.ncbi.nlm.nih.gov/pubmed/12383588). .

[80] *Rubin's Pathology - Clinicopathological Foundations of Medicine*. Maryland: Lippincott Williams & Wilkins. 2001. pp. 546. ISBN 0-7817-4733-3.

[81] Eichbaum FW. "'Wavy' myocardial fibers in spontaneous and experimental adrenergic cardiopathies" *Cardiology* 1975; **60**(6): 358–65. PMID 782705

[82] S Roy. Myocardial infarction (http://www.histopathology-india.net/Heart5.htm). Retrieved November 28, 2006.

[83] Fishbein MC. (1990). "Reperfusion injury". *Clin Cardiol* **13** (3): 213–7. doi:10.1152/ajpheart.00270.2002 (inactive 2008-06-25) . PMID 2182247 (http://www.ncbi.nlm.nih.gov/pubmed/2182247).

[84] Rossi S, editor. Australian Medicines Handbook 2006. Adelaide: Australian Medicines Handbook; 2006. ISBN 0-9757919-2-3.

[85] Smith A, Aylward P, Campbell T, *et al.* Therapeutic Guidelines: Cardiovascular, 4th edition. North Melbourne: Therapeutic Guidelines; 2003. ISSN 1327-9513

[86] Peters RJ, Mehta SR, Fox KA, Zhao F, Lewis BS, Kopecky SL, Diaz R, Commerford PJ, Valentin V, Yusuf S; Clopidogrel in Unstable angina to prevent Recurrent Events (CURE) Trial Investigators. (2003). "Effects of aspirin dose when used alone or in combination with clopidogrel in patients with acute coronary syndromes: observations from the Clopidogrel in Unstable angina to prevent Recurrent Events (CURE) study". *Circulation* **108** (14): 1682–7. doi: 10.1161/01.CIR.0000091201.39590.CB (http://dx.doi.org/10.1161/01.CIR.0000091201.39590.CB). PMID 14504182 (http://www.ncbi.nlm.nih.gov/pubmed/14504182).

[87] Yusuf S, Peto R, Lewis J, Collins R, Sleight P (1985). "Beta blockade during and after myocardial infarction: an overview of the randomized trials". *Prog Cardiovasc Dis* **27** (5): 335–71. doi: 10.1016/S0033-0620(85)80003-7 (http://dx.doi.org/10.1016/S0033-0620(85)80003-7). PMID 2858114 (http://www.ncbi.nlm.nih.gov/pubmed/2858114).

[88] Dargie HJ. (2001). "Effect of carvedilol on outcome after myocardial infarction in patients with left-ventricular dysfunction: the CAPRICORN randomised trial". *Lancet* **357** (9266): 1385–90. doi: 10.1016/S0140-6736(00)04560-8 (http://dx.doi.org/10.1016/S0140-6736(00)04560-8). PMID 11356434 (http://www.ncbi.nlm.nih.gov/pubmed/11356434).

[89] Pfeffer MA, Braunwald E, Moye LA, Basta L, Brown EJ Jr, Cuddy TE, Davis BR, Geltman EM, Goldman S, Flaker GC, et al. (1992). "Effect of captopril on mortality and morbidity in patients with left ventricular dysfunction after myocardial infarction. Results of the survival and ventricular enlargement trial. The SAVE Investigators". *N Engl J Med*. **327** (10): 669–77. PMID 1386652 (http://www.ncbi.nlm.nih.gov/pubmed/1386652).

[90] Sacks FM, Pfeffer MA, Moye LA, Rouleau JL, Rutherford JD, Cole TG, Brown L, Warnica JW, Arnold JM, Wun CC, Davis BR, Braunwald E. (1996). "The effect of pravastatin on coronary events after myocardial infarction in patients with average cholesterol levels. Cholesterol and Recurrent Events Trial investigators". *N Engl J Med* **335** (14): 1001–9. doi: 10.1056/NEJM199610033351401 (http://dx.doi.org/10.1056/NEJM199610033351401). PMID 8801446 (http://www.ncbi.nlm.nih.gov/pubmed/8801446).

[91] Sacks FM, Moye LA, Davis BR, Cole TG, Rouleau JL, Nash DT, Pfeffer MA, Braunwald E. (1998). "Relationship between plasma LDL concentrations during treatment with pravastatin and recurrent coronary events in the Cholesterol and Recurrent Events trial". *Circulation* **97** (15): 1446–52. PMID 9576424 (http://www.ncbi.nlm.nih.gov/pubmed/9576424).

[92] Ray KK, Cannon CP (2005). "The potential relevance of the multiple lipid-independent (pleiotropic) effects of statins in the management of acute coronary syndromes" (http://linkinghub.elsevier.com/retrieve/pii/S0735-1097(05)01773-0). *J. Am. Coll. Cardiol.* **46** (8): 1425–33. doi: 10.1016/j.jacc.2005.05.086 (http://dx.doi.org/10.1016/j.jacc.2005.05.086). PMID 16226165 (http://www.ncbi.nlm.nih.gov/pubmed/16226165). .

[93] Keating G, Plosker G (2004). "Eplerenone: a review of its use in left ventricular systolic dysfunction and heart failure after acute myocardial infarction". *Drugs* **64** (23): 2689–707. doi: 10.1157/13089615 (http://dx.doi.org/10.1157/13089615). PMID 15537370 (http://www.ncbi.nlm.nih.gov/pubmed/15537370).

[94] "Dietary supplementation with n-3 polyunsaturated fatty acids and vitamin E after myocardial infarction: results of the GISSI-Prevenzione trial. Gruppo Italiano per lo Studio della Sopravvivenza nell'Infarto miocardico". *Lancet* **354** (9177): 447–55. 2001. doi: 10.1016/S0140-6736(99)07072-5 (http://dx.doi.org/10.1016/S0140-6736(99)07072-5). PMID 10465168 (http://www.ncbi.nlm.nih.gov/pubmed/10465168).

[95] Leaf A, Albert C, Josephson M, Steinhaus D, Kluger J, Kang J, Cox B, Zhang H, Schoenfeld D (2005). "Prevention of fatal arrhythmias in high-risk subjects by fish oil n-3 fatty acid intake" (http://circ.ahajournals.org/cgi/content/full/112/18/2762). *Circulation* **112** (18): 2762–8. doi: 10.1161/CIRCULATIONAHA.105.549527 (http://dx.doi.org/10.1161/CIRCULATIONAHA.105.549527). PMID 16267249 (http://www.ncbi.nlm.nih.gov/pubmed/16267249). .

[96] Brouwer IA, Zock PL, Camm AJ, Bocker D, Hauer RN, Wever EF, Dullemeijer C, Ronden JE, Katan MB, Lubinski A, Buschler H, Schouten EG; SOFA Study Group. (2006). "Effect of fish oil on ventricular tachyarrhythmia and death in patients with implantable cardioverter defibrillators: the Study on Omega-3 Fatty Acids and Ventricular Arrhythmia (SOFA) randomized trial". *JAMA* **295** (22): 2613–9. doi: 10.1001/jama.295.22.2613 (http://dx.doi.org/10.1001/jama.295.22.2613). PMID 16772624 (http://www.ncbi.nlm.nih.gov/pubmed/16772624).

[97] Raitt MH, Connor WE, Morris C, Kron J, Halperin B, Chugh SS, McClelland J, Cook J, MacMurdy K, Swenson R, Connor SL, Gerhard G, Kraemer DF, Oseran D, Marchant C, Calhoun D, Shnider R, McAnulty J. (2005). "Fish oil supplementation and risk of ventricular tachycardia and ventricular fibrillation in patients with implantable defibrillators: a randomized controlled trial". *JAMA* **293** (23): 2284–91. doi: 10.1001/jama.293.23.2884 (http://dx.doi.org/10.1001/jama.293.23.2884). PMID 15956633 (http://www.ncbi.nlm.nih.gov/pubmed/15956633).

[98] TIME IS MUSCLE TIME WASTED IS MUSCLE LOST (http://www.ehac.org/st-agnes/EHAC_LifeandDeath/TimeisMuscle.htm). Early Heart Attack Care, St. Agnes Healthcare. Retrieved November 29, 2006.

[99] Meine TJ, Roe MT, Chen AY, *et al.* (2005). "Association of intravenous morphine use and outcomes in acute coronary syndromes: results from the CRUSADE Quality Improvement Initiative" (http://linkinghub.elsevier.com/retrieve/pii/S0002870305001493). *Am Heart J* **149** (6): 1043–9. doi: 10.1016/j.ahj.2005.02.010 (http://dx.doi.org/10.1016/j.ahj.2005.02.010). PMID 15976786 (http://www.ncbi.nlm.nih.gov/pubmed/15976786). .

[100] ISIS-2 Collaborative group (1988). "Randomized trial of intravenous streptokinase, oral aspirin, both, or neither among 17,187 cases of suspected acute myocardial infarction: ISIS-2". *Lancet* **2** (8607): 349–60. PMID 2899772 (http://www.ncbi.nlm.nih.gov/pubmed/2899772).

[101] ISIS-1 Collaborative Group (1986). "Randomised trial of intravenous atenolol among 16 027 cases of suspected acute myocardial infarction: ISIS-1". *Lancet* **2** (8498): 57–66. PMID 2873379 (http://www.ncbi.nlm.nih.gov/pubmed/2873379).

[102] The TIMI Study Group (1989). "Comparison of invasive and conservative strategies after treatment with intravenous tissue plasminogen activator in acute myocardial infarction". *N Engl J Med* **320** (10): 618–27. PMID 2563896 (http://www.ncbi.nlm.nih.gov/pubmed/2563896).

[103] McCord J, Jneid H, Hollander JE, *et al.* (April 2008). "Management of cocaine-associated chest pain and myocardial infarction: a scientific statement from the American Heart Association Acute Cardiac Care Committee of the Council on Clinical Cardiology". *Circulation* **117** (14): 1897–907. doi: 10.1161/CIRCULATIONAHA.107.188950 (http://dx.doi.org/10.1161/CIRCULATIONAHA.107.188950). PMID 18347214 (http://www.ncbi.nlm.nih.gov/pubmed/18347214).

[104] Faxon DP. "Coronary interventions and their impact on post myocardial infarction survival." *Clin Cardiol* 2005; **28**(11 Suppl 1):I38-44. PMID 16450811

[105] Heart attack first aid (http://www.nlm.nih.gov/medlineplus/ency/article/000063.htm). MedlinePlus. Retrieved December 3, 2006.

[106] Act In Time to Heart Attack Signs (http://www.nhlbi.nih.gov/actintime/index.htm) - NHLBI. Retrieved December 13, 2006.

[107] Brown AL, Mann NC, Daya M, Goldberg R, Meischke H, Taylor J, Smith K, Osganian S, Cooper L. (2000). "Demographic, belief, and situational factors influencing the decision to utilize emergency medical services among chest pain patients. Rapid Early Action for Coronary Treatment (REACT) study". *Circulation* **102** (2): 173–8. PMID 10889127 (http://www.ncbi.nlm.nih.gov/pubmed/10889127).

[108] Antman EM, Anbe DT, Armstrong PW, Bates ER, Green LA, Hand M, Hochman JS, Krumholz HM, Kushner FG, Lamas GA, Mullany CJ, Ornato JP, Pearle DL, Sloan MA, Smith SC Jr (2004). "ACC/AHA guidelines for the management of patients with ST-elevation myocardial infarction: a report of the American College of Cardiology/American Heart Association Task Force on Practice Guidelines (Committee to Revise the 1999 Guidelines for the Management of Patients With Acute Myocardial Infarction)" (http://www.acc.org/qualityandscience/clinical/guidelines/stemi/Guideline1/index.htm). *J Am Coll Cardiol* **44** (3): 671–719. doi: 10.1016/j.jacc.2004.07.002 (http://dx.doi.org/10.1016/j.jacc.2004.07.002). PMID 15358045 (http://www.ncbi.nlm.nih.gov/pubmed/15358045). .

[109] Antman EM, Anbe DT, Armstrong PW, *et al.* (August 2004). "ACC/AHA guidelines for the management of patients with ST-elevation myocardial infarction--executive summary. A report of the American College of Cardiology/American Heart Association Task Force on Practice Guidelines (Writing Committee to revise the 1999 guidelines for the management of patients with acute myocardial infarction)". *J. Am. Coll. Cardiol.* **44** (3): 671–719. doi: 10.1016/j.jacc.2004.07.002 (http://dx.doi.org/10.1016/j.jacc.2004.07.002). PMID 15358045 (http://www.ncbi.nlm.nih.gov/pubmed/15358045).

[110] Morrow DA, Antman EM, Sayah A, *et al.* (July 2002). "Evaluation of the time saved by prehospital initiation of reteplase for ST-elevation myocardial infarction: results of The Early Retavase-Thrombolysis in Myocardial Infarction (ER-TIMI) 19 trial" (http://linkinghub.elsevier.

com/retrieve/pii/S0735109702019368). *J. Am. Coll. Cardiol.* **40** (1): 71–7. doi: 10.1016/S0735-1097(02)01936-8 (http://dx.doi.org/10. 1016/S0735-1097(02)01936-8). PMID 12103258 (http://www.ncbi.nlm.nih.gov/pubmed/12103258). .

[111] Morrison LJ, Verbeek PR, McDonald AC, Sawadsky BV, Cook DJ. (2000). "Mortality and prehospital thrombolysis for acute myocardial infarction: A meta-analysis" (http://jama.ama-assn.org/cgi/reprint/283/20/2686. pdf?ijkey=c72b289825a3fd6ace7545ef61cd70936485e7e1) (PDF). *JAMA* **283** (20): 2686–92. doi:10.1001/jama.283.20.2686 (inactive 2009-11-08) . PMID 10819952 (http://www.ncbi.nlm.nih.gov/pubmed/10819952). .

[112] Rokos IC, Larson DM, Henry TD, *et al.* (2006). "Rationale for establishing regional ST-elevation myocardial infarction receiving center (SRC) networks". *Am. Heart J.* **152** (4): 661–7. doi: 10.1016/j.ahj.2006.06.001 (http://dx.doi.org/10.1016/j.ahj.2006.06.001). PMID 16996830 (http://www.ncbi.nlm.nih.gov/pubmed/16996830).

[113] Moyer P, Feldman J, Levine J, *et al.* (June 2004). "Implications of the Mechanical (PCI) vs Thrombolytic Controversy for ST Segment Elevation Myocardial Infarction on the Organization of Emergency Medical Services: The Boston EMS Experience". *Crit Pathw Cardiol* **3** (2): 53–61. doi: 10.1097/01.hpc.0000128714.35330.6d (http://dx.doi.org/10.1097/01.hpc.0000128714.35330.6d). PMID 18340140 (http://www.ncbi.nlm.nih.gov/pubmed/18340140).

[114] Terkelsen CJ, Lassen JF, Nørgaard BL, *et al.* (April 2005). "Reduction of treatment delay in patients with ST-elevation myocardial infarction: impact of pre-hospital diagnosis and direct referral to primary percutanous coronary intervention". *Eur. Heart J.* **26** (8): 770–7. doi: 10.1093/eurheartj/ehi100 (http://dx.doi.org/10.1093/eurheartj/ehi100). PMID 15684279 (http://www.ncbi.nlm.nih.gov/pubmed/ 15684279).T

[115] Henry TD, Atkins JM, Cunningham MS, *et al.* (April 2006). "ST-segment elevation myocardial infarction: recommendations on triage of patients to heart attack centers: is it time for a national policy for the treatment of ST-segment elevation myocardial infarction?". *J. Am. Coll. Cardiol.* **47** (7): 1339–45. doi: 10.1016/j.jacc.2005.05.101 (http://dx.doi.org/10.1016/j.jacc.2005.05.101). PMID 16580518 (http:// www.ncbi.nlm.nih.gov/pubmed/16580518).

[116] Rokos I. and Bouthillet T., "The emergency medical systems-to-balloon (E2B) challenge: building on the foundations of the D2B Alliance," (http://www.stemisystems.org/PDF/STEMIsystems_issue2.pdf) *STEMI Systems*, Issue Two, May 2007. Accessed June 16, 2007.

[117] Cannon, Christopher (1999). *Management of acute coronary syndromes*. Totowa, NJ: Humana Press. ISBN 0-89603-552-2.

[118] Lee KL, Woodlief LH, Topol EJ, et al. "Predictors of 30-Day Mortality in the Era of Reperfusion for Acute Myocardial Infarction." *Circulation* 1995; **91**: 1659-1668. PMID 7882472

[119] Stone GW, Grines CL, Browne KF, et al. "Predictors of in-hospital and 6-month outcome after acute myocardial infarction in the reperfusion era: the Primary Angioplasty in Myocardial Infarction (PAMI) trail." *J Am Coll Cardiol* 1995; **25**: 370-377. PMID 14645641

[120] "Indications for fibrinolytic therapy in suspected acute myocardial infarction: collaborative overview of early mortality and major morbidity results from all randomised trials of more than 1000 patients. Fibrinolytic Therapy Trialists' (FTT) Collaborative Group." *Lancet* 1994; **343**(8893): 311-22. PMID 7905143

[121] Verheugt FW, Gersh BJ, Armstrong PW. "Aborted myocardial infarction: a new target for reperfusion therapy." *Eur Heart J* 2006; **27**(8): 901-4. PMID 16543251

[122] Boersma E, Maas AC, Deckers JW, Simoons ML. "Early thrombolytic treatment in acute myocardial infarction: reappraisal of the golden hour." *Lancet* 1996; **348** (9030): 771-5. PMID 8813982

[123] "Effects of tissue plasminogen activator and a comparison of early invasive and conservative strategies in unstable angina and non-Q-wave myocardial infarction. Results of the TIMI IIIB Trial. Thrombolysis in Myocardial Ischemia." *Circulation* 1994; **89** (4): 1545-56. PMID 8149520

[124] Hochman JS, Sleeper LA, Webb JG, Sanborn TA, White HD, Talley JD, Buller CE, Jacobs AK, Slater JN, Col J, McKinlay SM, LeJemtel TH. (1999). "Early revascularization in acute myocardial infarction complicated by cardiogenic shock. SHOCK Investigators. Should We Emergently Revascularize Occluded Coronaries for Cardiogenic Shock". *N Engl J Med* **341** (9): 625–34. doi: 10.1056/NEJM199908263410901 (http://dx.doi.org/10.1056/NEJM199908263410901). PMID 10460813 (http://www.ncbi.nlm.nih. gov/pubmed/10460813).

[125] White HD, Van de Werf FJ. "Thrombolysis for acute myocardial infarction.." *Circulation* 1998; **97** (16): 1632-46. PMID 9593569

[126] The GUSTO investigators (1993). "An international randomized trial comparing four thrombolytic strategies for acute myocardial infarction. The GUSTO investigators". *N Engl J Med* **329** (10): 673–82. doi: 10.1056/NEJM199309023291001 (http://dx.doi.org/10.1056/ NEJM199309023291001). PMID 8204123 (http://www.ncbi.nlm.nih.gov/pubmed/8204123).

[127] Sabatine MS, Morrow DA, Montalescot G, Dellborg M, Leiva-Pons JL, Keltai M, Murphy SA, McCabe CH, Gibson CM, Cannon CP, Antman EM, Braunwald E; Clopidogrel as Adjunctive Reperfusion Therapy (CLARITY)-Thrombolysis in Myocardial Infarction (TIMI) 28 Investigators. (2005). "Angiographic and clinical outcomes in patients receiving low-molecular-weight heparin versus unfractionated heparin in ST-elevation myocardial infarction treated with fibrinolytics in the CLARITY-TIMI 28 Trial". *Circulation* **112** (25): 3846–54. doi: 10.1161/CIRCULATIONAHA.105.595397 (http://dx.doi.org/10.1161/CIRCULATIONAHA.105.595397). PMID 16291601 (http:// www.ncbi.nlm.nih.gov/pubmed/16291601).

[128] Cowley MJ, Hastillo A, Vetrovec GW, Fisher LM, Garrett R, Hess ML. (1983). "Fibrinolytic effects of intracoronary streptokinase administration in patients with acute myocardial infarction and coronary insufficiency". *Circulation* **67** (5): 1031–8. PMID 6831667 (http:// www.ncbi.nlm.nih.gov/pubmed/6831667).

[129] Lourenco DM, Dosne AM, Kher A, Samama M. (1989). "Effect of standard heparin and a low molecular weight heparin on thrombolytic and fibrinolytic activity of single-chain urokinase plasminogen activator *in vitro*". *Thromb Haemost* **62** (3): 923–6. PMID 2556812 (http://

www.ncbi.nlm.nih.gov/pubmed/2556812).
[130] Van de Werf F, Vanhaecke J, de Geest H, Verstraete M, Collen D. (1986). "Coronary thrombolysis with recombinant single-chain urokinase-type plasminogen activator in patients with acute myocardial infarction". *Circulation* **74** (5): 1066–70. PMID 2429783 (http://www.ncbi.nlm.nih.gov/pubmed/2429783).
[131] Bode C, Schoenermark S, Schuler G, Zimmermann R, Schwarz F, Kuebler W. (1988). "Efficacy of intravenous prourokinase and a combination of prourokinase and urokinase in acute myocardial infarction". *Am J Cardiol* **61** (13): 971–4. doi:10.1016/0002-9149(88)90108-7 (http://dx.doi.org/10.1016/0002-9149(88)90108-7). PMID 2452564 (http://www.ncbi.nlm.nih.gov/pubmed/2452564).
[132] Boersma E, Maas AC, Deckers JW, Simoons ML. (1996). "Early thrombolytic treatment in acute myocardial infarction: reappraisal of the golden hour". *Lancet* **348** (9030): 771–5. doi: 10.1016/S0140-6736(96)02514-7 (http://dx.doi.org/10.1016/S0140-6736(96)02514-7). PMID 8813982 (http://www.ncbi.nlm.nih.gov/pubmed/8813982).
[133] LATE trial intestigatos. (1993). "Late Assessment of Thrombolytic Efficacy (LATE) study with alteplase 6-24 hours after onset of acute myocardial infarction". *Lancet* **342** (8874): 759–66. doi: 10.1016/0140-6736(93)91538-W (http://dx.doi.org/10.1016/0140-6736(93)91538-W). PMID 8103874 (http://www.ncbi.nlm.nih.gov/pubmed/8103874).
[134] Chesebro JH, Knatterud G, Roberts R, Borer J, Cohen LS, Dalen J, Dodge HT, Francis CK, Hillis D, Ludbrook P, et al. (1987). "Thrombolysis in Myocardial Infarction (TIMI) Trial, Phase I: A comparison between intravenous tissue plasminogen activator and intravenous streptokinase. Clinical findings through hospital discharge". *Circulation* **76** (1): 142–54. PMID 3109764 (http://www.ncbi.nlm.nih.gov/pubmed/3109764).
[135] Keeley EC, Boura JA, Grines CL. (2003). "Primary angioplasty versus intravenous thrombolytic therapy for acute myocardial infarction: a quantitative review of 23 randomised trials". *Lancet* **361** (9351): 13–20. doi: 10.1016/S0140-6736(03)12113-7 (http://dx.doi.org/10.1016/S0140-6736(03)12113-7). PMID 12517460 (http://www.ncbi.nlm.nih.gov/pubmed/12517460).
[136] Grines CL, Browne KF, Marco J, Rothbaum D, Stone GW, O'Keefe J, Overlie P, Donohue B, Chelliah N, Timmis GC, et al. (1993). "A comparison of immediate angioplasty with thrombolytic therapy for acute myocardial infarction. The Primary Angioplasty in Myocardial Infarction Study Group". *N Engl J Med* **328** (10): 673–9. doi: 10.1056/NEJM199303113281001 (http://dx.doi.org/10.1056/NEJM199303113281001). PMID 8433725 (http://www.ncbi.nlm.nih.gov/pubmed/8433725).
[137] The Global Use of Strategies to Open Occluded Coronary Arteries in Acute Coronary Syndromes (GUSTO IIb) Angioplasty Substudy Investigators. (1997). "A clinical trial comparing primary coronary angioplasty with tissue plasminogen activator for acute myocardial infarction". *N Engl J Med* **336** (23): 1621–8. doi: 10.1056/NEJM199706053362301 (http://dx.doi.org/10.1056/NEJM199706053362301). PMID 9173270 (http://www.ncbi.nlm.nih.gov/pubmed/9173270).
[138] Boersma E; The Primary Coronary Angioplasty vs. Thrombolysis Group. "Does time matter? A pooled analysis of randomized clinical trials comparing primary percutaneous coronary intervention and in-hospital fibrinolysis in acute myocardial infarction patients." *Eur Heart J* 2006; 27(7):779-88. PMID 16513663
[139] Rokos IC, Larson DM, Henry TD, et al.; "Rationale for establishing regional ST-elevation myocardial infarction receiving center (SRC) networks." *Am Heart J* 2006; **152**(4):661-7. PMID 16996830
[140] Bradley EH, Herrin J, Wang Y, Barton BA, Webster TR, Mattera JA, Roumanis SA, Curtis JP, Nallamothu BK, Magid DJ, McNamara RL, Parkosewich J, Loeb JM, Krumholz HM. "Strategies for reducing the door-to-balloon time in acute myocardial infarction." *N Engl J Med* 2006; **355**(22): 2308-20. PMID 17101617
[141] "D2B: An Alliance for Quality" (http://d2b.acc.org/). American College of Cardiology. 2006. . Retrieved April 15, 2007.
[142] De Villiers JS, Anderson T, McMeekin JD, et al.. (2007). "Expedited transfer for primary percutaneous coronary intervention: a program evaluation" (http://www.pubmedcentral.nih.gov/articlerender.fcgi?tool=pmcentrez&artid=1891117). *CMAJ* **176** (13): 1833–8. doi: 10.1503/cmaj.060902 (http://dx.doi.org/10.1503/cmaj.060902). PMID 17576980 (http://www.ncbi.nlm.nih.gov/pubmed/17576980).
[143] Aversano T et al.. (2002). "Thrombolytic therapy vs primary percutaneous coronary intervention for myocardial infarction in patients presenting to hospitals without on-site cardiac surgery: a randomized controlled trial". *JAMA* **287** (15): 1943–51. doi: 10.1001/jama.287.15.1943 (http://dx.doi.org/10.1001/jama.287.15.1943). PMID 11960536 (http://www.ncbi.nlm.nih.gov/pubmed/11960536).
[144] Grines CL, Cox DA, Stone GW, Garcia E, Mattos LA, Giambartolomei A, Brodie BR, Madonna O, Eijgelshoven M, Lansky AJ, O'Neill WW, Morice MC. (1999). "Coronary angioplasty with or without stent implantation for acute myocardial infarction. Stent Primary Angioplasty in Myocardial Infarction Study Group". *N Engl J Med* **341** (26): 1949–56. doi: 10.1056/NEJM199912233412601 (http://dx.doi.org/10.1056/NEJM199912233412601). PMID 10607811 (http://www.ncbi.nlm.nih.gov/pubmed/10607811).
[145] Brener SJ, Barr LA, Burchenal JE, Katz S, George BS, Jones AA, Cohen ED, Gainey PC, White HJ, Cheek HB, Moses JW, Moliterno DJ, Effron MB, Topol EJ. (1998). "Randomized, placebo-controlled trial of platelet glycoprotein IIb/IIIa blockade with primary angioplasty for acute myocardial infarction. ReoPro and Primary PTCA Organization and Randomized Trial (RAPPORT) Investigators". *Circulation* **98** (8): 734–41. PMID 9727542 (http://www.ncbi.nlm.nih.gov/pubmed/9727542).
[146] Tcheng JE, Kandzari DE, Grines CL, Cox DA, Effron MB, Garcia E, Griffin JJ, Guagliumi G, Stuckey T, Turco M, Fahy M, Lansky AJ, Mehran R, Stone GW; CADILLAC Investigators. (2003). "Benefits and risks of abciximab use in primary angioplasty for acute myocardial infarction: the Controlled Abciximab and Device Investigation to Lower Late Angioplasty Complications (CADILLAC) trial". *Circulation* **108** (11): 1316–23. doi: 10.1161/01.CIR.0000087601.45803.86 (http://dx.doi.org/10.1161/01.CIR.0000087601.45803.86). PMID 12939213 (http://www.ncbi.nlm.nih.gov/pubmed/12939213).

[147] Mukherjee, Debabrata (2006). *900 Questions: An Interventional Cardiology Board Review*. Lippincott Williams & Wilkins. ISBN 0781773490.

[148] Babaev A, Frederick PD, Pasta DJ, Every N, Sichrovsky T, Hochman JS (2005). "Trends in management and outcomes of patients with acute myocardial infarction complicated by cardiogenic shock" (http://jama.ama-assn.org/cgi/pmidlookup?view=long&pmid=16046651). *JAMA* **294** (4): 448–54. doi: 10.1001/jama.294.4.448 (http://dx.doi.org/10.1001/jama.294.4.448). PMID 16046651 (http://www.ncbi.nlm.nih.gov/pubmed/16046651). .

[149] Townsend, Courtney M.; Beauchamp D.R., Evers M.B., Mattox K.L. (2004). *Sabiston Textbook of Surgery - The Biological Basis of Modern Surgical Practice* (http://www.elsevier.com/wps/find/bookdescription.cws_home/701163/description#description). Philadelphia, Pennsylvania: Elsevier Saunders. pp. 1871. ISBN 0-7216-0409-9. .

[150] Kaul TK, Fields BL, Riggins SL, Dacumos GC, Wyatt DA, Jones CR (1995). "Coronary artery bypass grafting within 30 days of an acute myocardial infarction" (http://linkinghub.elsevier.com/retrieve/pii/0003497595001255). *Ann. Thorac. Surg.* **59** (5): 1169–76. doi: 10.1016/0003-4975(95)00125-5 (http://dx.doi.org/10.1016/0003-4975(95)00125-5). PMID 7733715 (http://www.ncbi.nlm.nih.gov/pubmed/7733715). .

[151] Creswell LL, Moulton MJ, Cox JL, Rosenbloom M (1995). "Revascularization after acute myocardial infarction" (http://linkinghub.elsevier.com/retrieve/pii/000349759500351K). *Ann. Thorac. Surg.* **60** (1): 19–26. PMID 7598589 (http://www.ncbi.nlm.nih.gov/pubmed/7598589). .

[152] White HD, Assmann SF, Sanborn TA, et al. (2005). "Comparison of percutaneous coronary intervention and coronary artery bypass grafting after acute myocardial infarction complicated by cardiogenic shock: results from the Should We Emergently Revascularize Occluded Coronaries for Cardiogenic Shock (SHOCK) trial" (http://circ.ahajournals.org/cgi/pmidlookup?view=long&pmid=16186436). *Circulation* **112** (13): 1992–2001. doi: 10.1161/CIRCULATIONAHA.105.540948 (http://dx.doi.org/10.1161/CIRCULATIONAHA.105.540948). PMID 16186436 (http://www.ncbi.nlm.nih.gov/pubmed/16186436). .

[153] Hochman JS, Sleeper LA, Webb JG, Dzavik V, Buller CE, Aylward P, Col J, White HD; SHOCK Investigators. (2006). "Early revascularization and long-term survival in cardiogenic shock complicating acute myocardial infarction" (http://www.pubmedcentral.nih.gov/articlerender.fcgi?tool=pmcentrez&artid=1782030). *JAMA* **295** (21): 2511–5. doi: 10.1001/jama.295.21.2511 (http://dx.doi.org/10.1001/jama.295.21.2511). PMID 16757723 (http://www.ncbi.nlm.nih.gov/pubmed/16757723). .

[154] Raja SG, Haider Z, Ahmad M, Zaman H (2004). "Saphenous vein grafts: to use or not to use?" (http://linkinghub.elsevier.com/retrieve/pii/S1443-9506(04)00140-4). *Heart Lung Circ* **13** (4): 403–9. doi: 10.1016/j.hlc.2004.04.004 (http://dx.doi.org/10.1016/j.hlc.2004.04.004). PMID 16352226 (http://www.ncbi.nlm.nih.gov/pubmed/16352226). .

[155] Hannan EL, Racz MJ, Walford G, et al. (2005). "Long-term outcomes of coronary-artery bypass grafting versus stent implantation" (http://content.nejm.org/cgi/pmidlookup?view=short&pmid=15917382&promo=ONFLNS19). *N. Engl. J. Med.* **352** (21): 2174–83. doi: 10.1056/NEJMoa040316 (http://dx.doi.org/10.1056/NEJMoa040316). PMID 15917382 (http://www.ncbi.nlm.nih.gov/pubmed/15917382). .

[156] Bourassa MG (2000). "Clinical trials of coronary revascularization: coronary angioplasty vs. coronary bypass grafting" (http://meta.wkhealth.com/pt/pt-core/template-journal/lwwgateway/media/landingpage.htm?issn=0268-4705&volume=15&issue=4&spage=281). *Curr. Opin. Cardiol.* **15** (4): 281–6. doi: 10.1097/00001573-200007000-00013 (http://dx.doi.org/10.1097/00001573-200007000-00013). PMID 11139092 (http://www.ncbi.nlm.nih.gov/pubmed/11139092). .

[157] Hlatky MA, Boothroyd DB, Melsop KA, et al. (2004). "Medical costs and quality of life 10 to 12 years after randomization to angioplasty or bypass surgery for multivessel coronary artery disease" (http://circ.ahajournals.org/cgi/pmidlookup?view=long&pmid=15451795). *Circulation* **110** (14): 1960–6. doi: 10.1161/01.CIR.0000143379.26342.5C (http://dx.doi.org/10.1161/01.CIR.0000143379.26342.5C). PMID 15451795 (http://www.ncbi.nlm.nih.gov/pubmed/15451795). .

[158] Echt DS, Liebson PR, Mitchell LB, Peters RW, Obias-Manno D, Barker AH, Arensberg D, Baker A, Friedman L, Greene HL, et al. (1991). "Mortality and morbidity in patients receiving encainide, flecainide, or placebo. The Cardiac Arrhythmia Suppression Trial". *N Engl J Med* **324** (12): 781–8. PMID 1900101 (http://www.ncbi.nlm.nih.gov/pubmed/1900101). .

[159] Waldo AL, Camm AJ, deRuyter H, Friedman PL, MacNeil DJ, Pauls JF, Pitt B, Pratt CM, Schwartz PJ, Veltri EP. (1996). "Effect of d-sotalol on mortality in patients with left ventricular dysfunction after recent and remote myocardial infarction. The SWORD Investigators. Survival With Oral d-Sotalol". *Lancet* **348** (9019): 7–12. doi: 10.1016/S0140-6736(96)02149-6 (http://dx.doi.org/10.1016/S0140-6736(96)02149-6). PMID 8691967 (http://www.ncbi.nlm.nih.gov/pubmed/8691967). .

[160] Julian DG, Camm AJ, Frangin G, Janse MJ, Munoz A, Schwartz PJ, Simon P. (1997). "Randomised trial of effect of amiodarone on mortality in patients with left-ventricular dysfunction after recent myocardial infarction: EMIAT. European Myocardial Infarct Amiodarone Trial Investigators". *Lancet* **349** (9053): 667–74. doi: 10.1016/S0140-6736(96)09145-3 (http://dx.doi.org/10.1016/S0140-6736(96)09145-3). PMID 9078197 (http://www.ncbi.nlm.nih.gov/pubmed/9078197). .

[161] Youngwith, Janice (2008-02-06). "Saving hearts in the air" (http://www.dailyherald.com/special/americanheartmonth/2008/index.asp?id=11). Dailyherald.com. . Retrieved 2008-06-12.

[162] Dowdall N. "Is there a doctor on the aircraft?' Top 10 in-flight medical emergencies." *BMJ* 2000; **321**(7272):1336-7. PMID 11090520. Full text at PMC: 1119071 (http://www.pubmedcentral.gov/articlerender.fcgi?tool=pmcentrez&artid=1119071)

[163] Life after a Heart Attack (http://www.nhlbi.nih.gov/health/dci/Diseases/HeartAttack/HeartAttack_LivingWith.html). U.S. National Heart, Lung and Blood Institute. Retrieved December 2, 2006.

[164] Trisha Macnair. Recovering after a heart attack (http://www.bbc.co.uk/health/conditions/heartattackrecovery1.shtml). BBC, December 2005. Retrieved December 2, 2006.

[165] "Classification of Drivers' Licenses Regulations" (http://www.gov.ns.ca/just/regulations/regs/mvclasdl.htm). Nova Scotia Registry of Regulations. May 24, 2000. . Retrieved April 22, 2007.
[166] " Heart Attack: Getting Back Into Your Life After a Heart Attack (http://familydoctor.org/002.xml)". American Academy of Family Physicians, updated March 2005. Retrieved December 4, 2006.
[167] Schachinger V, Erbs S, Elsasser A, Haberbosch W, Hambrecht R, Holschermann H, Yu J, Corti R, Mathey DG, Hamm CW, Suselbeck T, Assmus B, Tonn T, Dimmeler S, Zeiher AM; REPAIR-AMI Investigators (2006). "Intracoronary bone marrow-derived progenitor cells in acute myocardial infarction". *N Engl J Med* **355** (12): 1210–21. doi: 10.1056/NEJMoa060186 (http://dx.doi.org/10.1056/NEJMoa060186). PMID 16990384 (http://www.ncbi.nlm.nih.gov/pubmed/16990384).
[168] Christman KL, Lee RJ. "Biomaterials for the Treatment of Myocardial Infarction". *J Am Coll Cardiol* 2006; **48**(5): 907-13. PMID 16949479
[169] Canto JG, Shlipak MG, Rogers WJ, Malmgren JA, Frederick PD, Lambrew CT, Ornato JP, Barron HV, Kiefe CI. (2000). "Prevalence, clinical characteristics, and mortality among patients with myocardial infarction presenting without chest pain". *JAMA* **283** (24): 3223–9. doi: 10.1001/jama.283.24.3223 (http://dx.doi.org/10.1001/jama.283.24.3223). PMID 10866870 (http://www.ncbi.nlm.nih.gov/pubmed/10866870).
[170] Yip HK, Wu CJ, Chang HW, Wang CP, Cheng CI, Chua S, Chen MC. (2003). "Cardiac rupture complicating acute myocardial infarction in the direct percutaneous coronary intervention reperfusion era" (http://www.chestjournal.org/cgi/reprint/124/2/565.pdf) (PDF). *Chest* **124** (2): 565–71. doi: 10.1378/chest.124.2.565 (http://dx.doi.org/10.1378/chest.124.2.565). PMID 12907544 (http://www.ncbi.nlm.nih.gov/pubmed/12907544). .
[171] Becker RC, Gore JM, Lambrew C, Weaver WD, Rubison RM, French WJ, Tiefenbrunn AJ, Bowlby LJ, Rogers WJ. (1996). "A composite view of cardiac rupture in the United States National Registry of Myocardial Infarction". *J Am Coll Cardiol* **27** (6): 1321–6. doi: 10.1016/0735-1097(96)00008-3 (http://dx.doi.org/10.1016/0735-1097(96)00008-3). PMID 8626938 (http://www.ncbi.nlm.nih.gov/pubmed/8626938).
[172] Moreno R, Lopez-Sendon J, Garcia E, Perez de Isla L, Lopez de Sa E, Ortega A, Moreno M, Rubio R, Soriano J, Abeytua M, Garcia-Fernandez MA. (2002). "Primary angioplasty reduces the risk of left ventricular free wall rupture compared with thrombolysis in patients with acute myocardial infarction". *J Am Coll Cardiol* **39** (4): 598–603. doi: 10.1016/S0735-1097(01)01796-X (http://dx.doi.org/10.1016/S0735-1097(01)01796-X). PMID 11849857 (http://www.ncbi.nlm.nih.gov/pubmed/11849857).
[173] Shin P, Sakurai M, Minamino T, Onishi S, Kitamura H. (1983). "Postinfarction cardiac rupture. A pathogenetic consideration in eight cases". *Acta Pathol Jpn* **33** (5): 881–93. PMID 6650169 (http://www.ncbi.nlm.nih.gov/pubmed/6650169).
[174] Podrid, Philip J.; Peter R. Kowey (2001). *Cardiac Arrhythmia: Mechanisms, Diagnosis, and Management*. Lippincott Williams & Wilkins. ISBN 0781724864.
[175] Sung, Ruey J.; Michael R. Lauer (2000). *Fundamental Approaches to the Management of Cardiac Arrhythmias*. Springer. ISBN 0792365593.
[176] Josephson, Mark E. (2002). *Clinical Cardiac Electrophysiology: Techniques and Interpretations*. Lippincott Williams & Wilkins. ISBN 0683306936.
[177] Lopez de Sa E, Lopez-Sendon J, Anguera I, Bethencourt A, Bosch X; Proyecto de Estudio del Pronostico de la Angina (PEPA) Investigators. "Prognostic value of clinical variables at presentation in patients with non-ST-segment elevation acute coronary syndromes: results of the Proyecto de Estudio del Pronostico de la Angina (PEPA)." *Medicine (Baltimore)* 2002; **81**(6): 434-42. PMID 12441900
[178] Krumholz H *et al*. "Patterns of hospital performance in acute myocardial infarction and heart failure - 30-day mortality and readmission" (http://circoutcomes.ahajournals.org/cgi/content/abstract/CIRCOUTCOMES.109.883256v1). *Circulation: Cardiovascular Quality and Outcomes*. doi: 10.1161/CIRCOUTCOMES.109.883256 (http://dx.doi.org/10.1161/CIRCOUTCOMES.109.883256). .
[179] Fox KA, Dabbous OH, Goldberg RJ, Pieper KS, Eagle KA, Van de Werf F, Avezum A, Goodman SG, Flather MD, Anderson FA Jr, Granger CB. "Prediction of risk of death and myocardial infarction in the six months after presentation with acute coronary syndrome: prospective multinational observational study (GRACE)." *BMJ* 2006; **333**(7578):1091. PMID 17032691
[180] Weir RA, McMurray JJ, Velazquez EJ. (2006). "Epidemiology of heart failure and left ventricular systolic dysfunction after acute myocardial infarction: prevalence, clinical characteristics, and prognostic importance". *Am J Cardiol* **97** (10A): 13F–25F. doi: 10.1016/j.amjcard.2006.03.005 (http://dx.doi.org/10.1016/j.amjcard.2006.03.005). PMID 16698331 (http://www.ncbi.nlm.nih.gov/pubmed/16698331).
[181] Bosch X, Theroux P. (2005). "Left ventricular ejection fraction to predict early mortality in patients with non-ST-segment elevation acute coronary syndromes". *Am Heart J* **150** (2): 215–20. doi: 10.1016/j.ahj.2004.09.027 (http://dx.doi.org/10.1016/j.ahj.2004.09.027). PMID 16086920 (http://www.ncbi.nlm.nih.gov/pubmed/16086920).
[182] Nicod P, Gilpin E, Dittrich H, Polikar R, Hjalmarson A, Blacky A, Henning H, Ross J (1989). "Short- and long-term clinical outcome after Q wave and non-Q wave myocardial infarction in a large patient population". *Circulation* **79** (3): 528–36. PMID 2645061 (http://www.ncbi.nlm.nih.gov/pubmed/2645061).
[183] Liew R, Sulfi S, Ranjadayalan K, Cooper J, Timmis AD. (2006). "Declining case fatality rates for acute myocardial infarction in South Asian and white patients in the past 15 years" (http://www.pubmedcentral.nih.gov/articlerender.fcgi?tool=pmcentrez&artid=1861115). *Heart* **92** (8): 1030–4. doi: 10.1136/hrt.2005.078634 (http://dx.doi.org/10.1136/hrt.2005.078634). PMID 16387823 (http://www.ncbi.nlm.nih.gov/pubmed/16387823).
[184] "Cause of Death - UC Atlas of Global Inequality" (http://ucatlas.ucsc.edu/cause.php). Center for Global, International and Regional Studies (CGIRS) at the University of California Santa Cruz. . Retrieved December 7, 2006.

[185] "Deaths and percentage of total death for the 10 leading causes of death: United States, 2002-2003" (http://www.cdc.gov/nchs/data/hestat/leadingdeaths03_tables.pdf) (PDF). National Center of Health Statistics. . Retrieved April 17, 2007.
[186] Mukherjee AK. (1995). "Prediction of coronary heart disease using risk factor categories". *J Indian Med Assoc* **93** (8): 312–5. PMID 8713248 (http://www.ncbi.nlm.nih.gov/pubmed/8713248).
[187] Ghaffar A, Reddy KS and Singhi M (2004). "Burden of non-communicable diseases in South Asia" (http://www.bmj.com/cgi/reprint/328/7443/807.pdf) (PDF). *BMJ* **328** (7443): 807–810. doi: 10.1136/bmj.328.7443.807 (http://dx.doi.org/10.1136/bmj.328.7443.807). PMID 15070638 (http://www.ncbi.nlm.nih.gov/pubmed/15070638). PMC 383378 (http://www.pubmedcentral.nih.gov/articlerender.fcgi?tool=pmcentrez&artid=383378). .
[188] Rastogi T, Vaz M, Spiegelman D, Reddy KS, Bharathi AV, Stampfer MJ, Willett WC and Ascheriol A (2004). "Physical activity and risk of coronary heart disease in India" (http://ije.oxfordjournals.org/cgi/reprint/33/4/759.pdf) (PDF). *Int. J. Epidemiol* **33** (4): 1–9. doi: 10.1093/ije/dyh042 (http://dx.doi.org/10.1093/ije/dyh042). PMID 15044412 (http://www.ncbi.nlm.nih.gov/pubmed/15044412). .
[189] Gupta R. (2007). "Escalating Coronary Heart Disease and Risk Factors in South Asians" (http://indianheartjournal.com/editorial007.pdf) (PDF). *Indian Heart Journal*: 214–17. .
[190] Gupta R, Misra A, Pais P, Rastogi P and Gupta VP. (2006). "Correlation of regional cardiovascular disease mortality in India with lifestyle and nutritional factors" (http://www.sciencedirect.com/science?_ob=MImg&_imagekey=B6T16-4GFV5CY-4-3&_cdi=4882&_user=209690&_orig=search&_coverDate=04/14/2006&_sk=998919996&view=c&wchp=dGLzVlz-zSkzV&md5=050edf99a813f475b985c8d590c86228&ie=/sdarticle.pdf) (PDF). *International Journal of Cardiology* **108** (3): 291–300. doi: 10.1016/j.ijcard.2005.05.044 (http://dx.doi.org/10.1016/j.ijcard.2005.05.044). PMID 15978684 (http://www.ncbi.nlm.nih.gov/pubmed/15978684). .
[191] Workers' Compensation FAQ (http://www.pvamu.edu/pages/2026.asp). Prairie View A&M University. Retrieved November 22, 2006.
[192] SIGNIFICANT DECISIONS Subject Index (http://www.biia.wa.gov/significantdecisions/contents.htm). Board of Industrial Insurance Appeals. Retrieved November 22, 2006.
[193] http://www.americanheart.org/heartattack
[194] http://www.nlm.nih.gov/medlineplus/heartattack.html
[195] http://hp2010.nhlbihin.net/atpiii/calculator.asp?usertype=pub

Article Sources and Contributors

Kawasaki disease *Source*: http://en.wikipedia.org/w/index.php?oldid=339797614 *Contributors*: ASLTerp, Ageekgal, AkiAkira, Alansohn, Alhth, Amerindianarts, Andri Egilsson, Arcadian, Arimareiji, Atlas87, Axl, Azzyjr, BlueLint, Bobet, Brendanconway, CO, Calmer Waters, Captain Seafort, Ched Davis, Cherubino, Chwats, CopperKettle, Davidruben, DeadEyeArrow, Delirium, Djsincla, Doc United States, Draeco, Dreadpiratetif, DropDeadGorgias, Drumex, Durova, EBY3221, Eearhartt, Ejl, El C, F W Nietzsche, Fabrictramp, Falcon8765, Francis Tyers, Frank, Fuzbaby, G-J, GBizzle, Gadfium, Gkanai, Gladys j cortez, GngstrMNKY, Grandmasterka, GregorB, Gregorius Pilosus, Grendelkhan, HelloAnnyong, Hu12, Immunize, Iridescent, J.delanoy, J04n, JamesAM, Jamesfuhrman, Jellonuts, Jetman, Jfdwolff, Jmh649, Junkyardprince, Jynx980, Kea2, Kilbad, Laurencq, Lights33, Lisarieden, Lisatwo, Lycanthrope, Marchije, Martin451, Medmaxo, Mishalak, Missmimi, Muijz, Nbauman, NeoDeGenero, Netkinetic, Newportm, No Guru, Ntsimp, Nuno Tavares, Oda Mari, Ohnoitsjamie, Orlandoturner, PEHowland, Paste, Pdeitiker, Pinball22, Pkoetters, Purplefreaks, RedArrow21, Rich Farmbrough, Rohh, Rumiton, Sainandfable, Sinneed, Sturm55, The Parting Glass, The Thing That Should Not Be, Timcs01, Tomtheman5, Trcunning, Unyoyega, W guice, Werdan7, WhisperToMe, Wkrocek, Wouterstomp, Wwallacee, Yosri, ZayZayEM, Пипумбрик, דוד55, 224 anonymous edits

Skin *Source*: http://en.wikipedia.org/w/index.php?oldid=339588811 *Contributors*: *drew, 194.78.109.xxx, 3dscience, 7, 914ian915, A suyash, AB, Aaron Brenneman, Accuruss, AdamJacobMuller, Ahoerstemeier, Aitias, Alansohn, Albrozdude, Alexey Feldgendler, Alexfusco5, AlexiusHoratius, Algirdas, Ali, Aliciacahill, Alliecat96, Allstarecho, Anaxial, Anclation, Anders Torlind, Andre Engels, Andrewtn, Andy Marchbanks, Andycjp, Andymac345, Angela, Anlace, Anonymous3190, Antandrus, Arcadian, Arielco, ArmadilloFromHell, Arteitle, Aryangarg, Ash231, AshLin, Ashadeofgrey, Atif.t2, Atomaton, Atosecond, Aujlakam, AxelBoldt, Baboon Faceless, Backslash Forwardslash, Ballista, Barek, Barneca, Barticus88, Basharh, Beano, Bettia, Bhadani, Bhamv, BiT, Bilbillbilll, BobKawanaka, Bobo192, Bogey97, Bomac, Bongwarrior, BoomerAB, Bradley1992, BrianKnez, Brianga, Brillig20, BrokenSphere, Bryonbrock, Bubbleboy2000, Bubblebutt2, C+C, CSWarren, Caltas, Can't sleep, clown will eat me, Canaima, Capricorn42, Capt. James T. Kirk, Captain panda, Carax, Ccalvin, Cdang, Cdonaltc, CerealBabyMilk, Charles Sturm, Charley white, Chefyingi, ChemGardener, ChrisCork, Chrislk02, Clawed, Cocoaguy, Codycod10, Colin Pomeroy, CommonsDelinker, Conversion script, Cooljuno411, CryptoDerk, Cuntvaginal, Da monster under your bed, Dan East, DanP, Danelo, Dante Alighieri, DarthVader, DaughterofSun, David Schaich, David Stewart, DavidWBrooks, Davidovic, Davidruben, Davidwr, Dawnseeker2000, Dbachmann, Deli nk, Delldot, DennyColt, Deolankar, DerHexer, Dethme0w, Diberri, Digitalgadget, Dina, Dionnica, Discospinster, DivineAlpha, Djsasso, Docflash, Donald Albury, Donarreiskoffer, Doubletrouble2000, Dragana666, Drawnedlac, Dreg743, Drgnu23, Dysprosia, Ebricca, Ed Fitzgerald, Editorofthewiki, Eelin33, Eleassar777, Elkost, Emezei, Emmanuelm, Emote, Emptymountains, Enauspeaker, Enigmaman, Enochlau, Enzo Aquarius, Epbr123, Eras-mus, Esanchez7587, Escape Orbit, Eu.stefan, Eubanks718, Evil saltine, Ewlyahoocom, Excirial, Faithlessthewonderboy, Faradayplank, Felizdenovo, Fences and windows, Fiilott, Filipop, Firsfron, Fish and karate, Forschung, Fratrep, Fredrik, Freecat, FritzG, Fsotrain09, Fuzzform, Gambit5639, Ged3000, Giftlite, GlassCobra, Glen, Glimz, Gogo Dodo, Goodnightmush, Goodthroughout, GraemeL, Grafen, Gurch, Gurubrahma, Gwernol, HalfShadow, Heiland.alex, Heliac, Henry1245, Herd of Swine, Heron, HexaChord, Hgamboa, Hirohisat, HI540511, Hollgor, Hoof Hearted, Horselover Frost, IRP, Iamtheactor, Iancarter, Inferno, Lord of Penguins, InfoCan, Inge-Lyubov, Inky, Instinct, Inter16, Irishguy, It Is Me Here, Ithunn, J.delanoy, J04n, JNW, JSmith60, JYolkowski, Jac16888, Jack324, Jake Wartenberg, Jauerback, Jay-mob, Jdavidb, JeffreyN, Jennavecia, JeremyA, Jersey emt, Jfdwolff, JinJian, Jlittlet, Jllax154321, Jmoney45, Jmundo, Joehall45, JohnOwens, Jojhutton, Jordan Yang, Jusdafax, KCinDC, Kaiba, Kalamkaar, Kandar, Kaobear, Katalaveno, Kazvorpal, Keenan Pepper, Ketsuekigata, Kgasso, Kilbad, King of Hearts, Kirachinmoku, Kku, Knowledge Seeker, KnowledgeOfSelf, Korg, Kse319, Kurzydesignf1, Kyle1278, LFlippyl, LauraOrganaSolo, Leevanjackson, Lightmouse, Lights, Liliya0323, Lir, LittleHow, LittleOldMe, Llort, Llydawr, Loren.wilton, Lradrama, Lucky Mitch, Luk, Luka Krstulović, Luke the fluke, Luna Santin, LynnS, MC10, MER-C, MK8, Mainpush, Maitch, Man vyi, Mani1, Maplestorywiki123, Marco Krohn, Marcus Brute, Marnanel, Martin451, Marxmanster, Mattbrundage, Matthew Yeager, Maxim, Maxis ftw, Mayooranathan, McSly, Mcorazao, Mdanciu, MeMeMe789, Meske, Mets501, Mhking, Michael Hardy, Mikael Häggström, Mike2vil, Mitch Ames, Mjmcm, Monkeyman, Moonriddengirl, Moyogo, Mr. Lefty, MrFish, MrOllie, MrSpectacles, Mrdebeuker, Mrdice, MuZemike, Myanw, Mygerardromance, MysteryDog, NHRHS2010, NPTV, Nakon, Naohiro19 revertvandal, NawlinWiki, Nburden, Neelix, NeilN, NellieBly, Neparis, NewEnglandYankee, Newfoundlander, Newknwldg 76, Ngb, Nick C, NickBush24, NickelShoe, Nihiltres, Nihlibrary, NikkiK90, Ninebyzero, Nishkid64, Nsaa, Nunquam Dormio, Nutriveg, Oatmeal batman, October skies blue, Oda Mari, Ohnoitsjamie, Ojigiri, Olaffpomona, Oleg Alexandrov, Oliphaunt, OllieFury, Omegatron, Opabinia regalis, Ossmann, OverlordQ, Oysterguitarist, Palica, Patrick, Paul August, Pearle, Perey, Perrydeath, Peter L, Philip Trueman, Phoenix-wiki, Phoenix79, Physicsguy891, Piano non troppo, PinchasC, Pinethicket, Pinkadelica, Pit, Plm209, Poor Yorick, Porqin, Prashanthns, PrestonH, Pseudomonas, Psinu, PurpleZone2000, Qaz, Qmfosejs, Quaeler, QueenCake, R, RainbowOfLight, Razimantv, Recognizance, Renaissancee, Rettetast, RexNL, Rhs1980, Rhys, Riandavis, Riversider2008, Rob Hooft, Robert K S, RodC, Rodsan18, Rooji11, Rsabbatini, Runefrost, S, SJP, Sabbut, Saimhe, Saintly, Samsara, Sarc37, Saxmanrox, Scandinaviantranslator, Sceptre, SchfiftyThree, Sciurinæ, Scottalter, Sdw25, Secretlondon, Sefuerte, Senorpueblo, Shadiac, Sharkface217, Shoeofdeath, SimonP, Sintaku, Sionus, Skunkboy74, Sl, Slakr, Smalljim, Smokizzy, Smooth O, Snek01, Snowolf, Sodium, Sotakeit, Spaully, Spitfire, Spylab, Squirt2711, StaticGull, Stephenb, Steven0195, Subash.chandran007, Sugarcubez, SuperHamster, Svedectvi, Swarm, Sylent, Sysy, Tariqabjotu, Tearfate, TeddyA.i., Template namespace initialisation script, TenOfAllTrades, Texture, ThatWikiGuy, Thatguyflint, The Anome, The Arbiter, The High Fin Sperm Whale, The Thing That Should Not Be, The wub, Thedavester, Thedjatclubrock, Thegreatdr, Thinboy00, Thucydides of Thrace, Tiddly Tom, Tide rolls, Tim1357, Timir2, Tj21, Tlcookcarney, Tom harrison, Tombomp, Tony K10, Tpicompany, TravelinSista, Trevor MacInnis, Tristanb, Twsx, Typer 525, USANational, Ukexpat, Uxiwu, VN503, Vary, Vaux, Vector Potential, Veinor, Versageek, Vicarious, Vikramg19, Vinayshukla89, Vishnava, Voyagerfan5761, Vsion, W.Ross, WLU, Watchtradition, Werdan7, Werdna, WhatamIdoing, Whipoorwill, Whiskey in the Jar, WikHead, Wiki alf, Wikid77, Wikidudeman, WikipedianMarlith, Will Blake, WillMcC, Willking1979, Willtron, Wimt, Winchelsea, Wouterstomp, Wyatt915, Xenure, Xy7, Yvwv, Zackalak74, Zandperl, Zaphod-Swe, Åkebråke, Александър, Саша Стефановић, 1106 anonymous edits

Mucous membrane *Source*: http://en.wikipedia.org/w/index.php?oldid=334578342 *Contributors*: Andre Engels, Andrea105, Andrewin, Antandrus, Anthony Appleyard, Arcadian, Arcadie, Arkwatem, Arnold Layne had a Strange Hobby, Aua, Bevo, Bobo192, CUSENZA Mario, Carcharoth, Carpentc, Cgingold, Ckelsh, Cool3, David.Monniaux, Delldot, Drgarden, EdPage, Exigence, Fishtobird, Gerrish, Gurch, Hans Adler, Hugh7, InvictaHOG, Isidore, JFreeman, Jaknouse, Japanese Searobin, JohnOwens, Jonathan.s.kt, KarlM, Kenyon, King of Hearts (old account 2), Leal Nightrunner, LordK, Mani1, Matt Deres, Maxxicum, Minimac94, Pjvpjv, Renato Caniatti, Reytan, RuM, Sardanaphalus, Schrandit, SimonP, Snigbrook, Snowmanradio, Souad27, TheEgyptian, TheLimbicOne, Timwi, Velho, Vinay, Wisebridge, Wknight94, X1987x, 82 anonymous edits

Lymph node *Source*: http://en.wikipedia.org/w/index.php?oldid=339191834 *Contributors*: Abd, Ahanes, Aitias, Allstarecho, Andbir, Ann jeena, Arcadian, Arpingstone, AstroHurricane001, AtmanDave, Avono, Aworra, Bball4eva13, Beano, Bear475, Beetstra, BillySharps, Blindman shady, Bobo192, Bongwarrior, Bramio, Breath-relic, Brim, Bryan Derksen, CJMomo, CanDo, CanadianLinuxUser, Catgut, Chiaotzu87, Cholmes75, Chrysaor, Cje, Cometstyles, CommonsDelinker, Crownjewel82, Ctmt, DHeyward, Da monster under your bed, DabMachine, Danierrr, Daughter of Mímir, Demosn01, Deskana, Dessymona, Diberri, DocWatson42, Doczilla, Dontbeaschmuck, DopefishJustin, DragonHawk, Drgnu23, Dysepsion, Eeekster, Eleassar, Epbr123, Erkcan, FeRD NYC, Feyer, Foobar, Frmoraes, Funky Monkey, Fuzzform, Gansxcore, Giftlite, Golbez, GraYoshi2x, Haakon, Hardyplants, Hennessey, Patrick, Herophilus, Horsten, Hu12, Huckfinne, Ida Shaw, Indon, Insanity Incarnate, J.delanoy, Japanese Searobin, Jeremykemp, Jfdwolff, Jklin, Jmvalin, Josh Parris, Junafani, Junglo, KC Panchal, Kantokano, Kfc1864, Kntrabssi, Koshatul, Kostisl, Kuru, Kwamikagami, Laurascudder, LearnAnatomy, Lennert B, Lews Therin, Light current, Lingosalad, LizardJr8, Luk, Lymphoma, MPerel, Mani1, MarcoTolo, Mathrick, Mauvila, MaxSem, Mboedick, Mboverload, Mecanismo, Mikael Häggström, Mike Rosoft, Mike2vil, Mimihitam, Monkeyman, NSR, Nadav1, Naniwako, Nephron, Neverquick, Nicholas Perkins, Nmg20, Not Incompetent, Nsaa, Obli, Osm agha, PDH, Patxi Iurra, Pit, Quinsareth, R0, Ran, Rasmus Faber, Renato Caniatti, Rjwilmsi, Robert McClenon, Rod57, Roo72, SCA Bulgaria, Salvor, Sbuckley, Secretlondon, Serephine, Sfmammamia, Skier Dude, Snoyes, SpaceFlight89, Speaking array, SpuriousQ, Stephan Leeds, StephenTreacy, Tapir Terrific, Template namespace initialisation script, TexasAndroid, Thingg, Thumperward, ToNToNi, TomikB, Tsemii, Tvarnoe, Twilight Realm, Uwe Gille, Vanished188, Vegetator, Voodoodolphins, WBardwin, Wdustbuster, Whiner01, Wikieditor06, Wildcat156, Wimt, WmGB, Wouterstomp, X201, YUL89YYZ, Yamamoto Ichiro, Yopure, سمرقندی, 370 anonymous edits

Blood vessel *Source*: http://en.wikipedia.org/w/index.php?oldid=338249606 *Contributors*: Air Bear, Alansohn, Alex Batt, Alex.tan, Alpha 4615, Alphachimp, Andre Engels, Andrew 1212, Annemo, Anonymous Dissident, Antandrus, Arcadian, Auxiliary Watchlist, BarretBonden, Bcatt, Bensaccount, Beve, Bfigura's puppy, Bomac, Bongat122, Chasingsol, Chromaticity, Closedmouth, Cremepuff222, Darth Mike, Deor, DerHexer, Diderot's dreams, Discospinster, Drgarden, ENGMED, Edgar181, ElinorD, Ellomate, Ellywa, EnSamulili, Eric-Wester, Everyking, Figma, Fritzpoll, Fromgermany, GTBacchus, Gggh, Hovea, Ianthegecko, Insomniduck, Irving92, Ixfd64, J.delanoy, JForget, JSpung, James086, Jdrewitt, Jfdwolff, Julesd, Jóna Þórunn, Keegan, Kerotan, Kieff, Kingjalis1, Knutux, Kosebamse, Kyle1278, LAX, LadyofHats, Lahroo, Lambmeat, Liftarn, Lipothymia, Lova Falk, Luna Santin, MAlvis, MER-C, Macy, Malinaccier, Mamyles, Marek69, Master of Puppets, Mentifisto, Merube 89, Michael K. Edwards, Mintleaf, Mote, Neutrality, NickGorton, Njmagnusson, Nomad2u001, Nuno Tavares, Orange Chicken7875, PFHLai, PhatRita, Qxz, Rob Hooft, Rsvpair, RuM, Sander123, SarekOfVulcan, Sasuke Sarutobi, Scarian, Shanes, Sigmamax, Sliggy, Smalljim, Smithbrenon, Someone else, Sopoforic, Svetlana Miljkovic, Tabletop, Taranet, Template namespace initialisation script, The Thing That Should Not Be, The man3001, Tresiden, Troop350, Tuxide, Unschool, Utcursch, Vary, Vishnava, VvV, Wavelength, Wikieditor06, Wikivmk, WojPob, World, XJamRastafire, Yamamoto Ichiro, Zack wadghiri, Ziga, 287 anonymous edits

Tomisaku Kawasaki *Source*: http://en.wikipedia.org/w/index.php?oldid=339799438 *Contributors*: Alison9, Arcadian, Atouchofgreydotca, Ichiro Kikuchi, RP88, Redf0x, Synergy, TonyW, 2 anonymous edits

Heart *Source*: http://en.wikipedia.org/w/index.php?oldid=340067998 *Contributors*: *crups*, 16@r, 210.50.203.xxx, 2enable, 2v11, 334a, 3dscience, A. B., A8UDI, AHands, Aaron Brenneman, Abcmmmm, Abonilla, Academic Challenger, Accarpenter, Adam7davies, Adambro, Adashiel, Adi4094, AdjustShift, Ae77, Aetylus, Aff123a, AgentPeppermint, Agüeybaná, Ahoerstemeier, Aka042, Akanemoto, Aksi great, Alansohn, Alberto Orlandini, Alesnormales, Alex.tan, AlexandKevin, Alexius08, AlexiusHoratius, Alexyu1, Algormortis, Alison, AliveFreeHappy, Alpha 4615, Alpha Omicron, Alphachimp, Altenmann, Alucardxt, AmiDaniel, Amicon, Amplitude101, Anaxial, Andr987, Andre Engels, Andrea105, AndreasPraefcke, Andrewa, Andrewpmk, Andy85719, AndyZ, Andycjp, Anetode, Angela, AngryParsley, Anirvan, Anjelelsy, Anonymi, Anonymous101, Anonymousboy04, Antandrus, Antonio Lopez, Ap, Apokryltaros, Arakunem, Arbitrarily0, Arcadian, Arcenciel, ArielGold, Arun Philip, Aryeh, Asaunders135, Ascorbic, Asterion, AstroPig7, Astronaut97, Atomic Cosmos, AuburnPilot, Avono, AxelBoldt, Ayla, Az1568, AzaToth, Babyblack, Backslash Forwardslash, Barfooz, Baseball Bugs, Baswellbrat408, Batman n' robin, Beetstra, Benpayne2004, Bensaccount, Bernard the Varanid, BesselDekker, Bhadani, BigBadUglyBugFacedBabyEatingO'Brian, Bigboithecoolest, BillyWagner13BS, Bisqwit, Biŋhai, BjarteSorensen, Bkonrad, Blanchardb, BlueAg09, Bluezy, Bmicomp, Bob f it, Bobbo, Bobdoc, Bobisbob, Bobo192, Bobthesmall, Bogey97, Bomac, Bomberzboy, Bongwarrior, Bookfairy12, Bradjamesbrown, Brandmeister, Brim, Brusegadi, Bryan Derksen, Bth, Bubbyreallystinks,

Burntsauce, Bushcarrot, Caesura, Calco blue, Calebe, California123123, Calor, Caltas, Can't sleep, clown will eat me, Canderson7, CanisRufus, Capricorn42, Cardiac Morph, CardinalDan, Carlsotr, Carlwev, Caspian, Catgut, Cbrown1023, Cburnett, Cd.dolata, Celithemis, Chaldor, Chasingsol, Cheddon, Chris bonney, Christal1999, CliffC, Closedmouth, Cmichael, Coatbutton, Coffee, Cogorno, Cometstyles, CommonsDelinker, Computer 3, Computer66, Cornucopia, CplHare992, CptUnconscious, Craig9000, Cremepuff222, Curps, Cxz111, Cyktsui, D Dinneen, D6, DJ Clayworth, DVD R W, Da monster under your bed, Dadude3320, Dalillama, Damicatz, DanD, Danny beaudoin, Dantecubed, Dark jedi requiem, Darth Panda, DaveJ7, David Henderson, DavidCary, DavidHolden, Davidsfarm, Dawnseeker2000, Dcfleck, Deadly Dozen, Deconstructhis, Deeptrivia, Delirium, Delldot, Demoish, DerHexer, Derg999, Dfrg.msc, Dgonzalezz62, Dhollm, Diberri, Dina, Discospinster, Dissident, Doctor11, Dodiad, Dominics Fire, Dorftrottel, DoubleBlue, Dougofborg, Doulos Christos, Dpbsmith, Drakebiologylaboratory, Dreadstar, Drewthedude, Drini, Drivenapart, Drmies, Droid392, Drypelia, DuBose, Dungodung, Dureo, Dynaflow, E!, ESkog, EarthPerson, Ebyabe, Ec5618, Ed g2s, Edsuom, Edward321, Effeietsanders, Either way, Ejay, ElBeeroMan, Eleassar777, Elkman, Enchanter, Endomorphic, Epbr123, Epingchris, Epolk, Erdal Ronahi, Eribro, Eric Kvaalen, Ericamick, Erik9, Esanchez7587, Etruria, Eu.stefan, Eubanks718, Eukesh, Evercat, Everyking, Evil Monkey, Excirial, FaerieInGrey, Faggyass17, Fahadsadah, Fairychild, Faithlessthewonderboy, Faradayplank, Farosdaughter, Farside, Fastily, Favonian, Felyza, FetchcommsAWB, Fharper1961, FiP, Fieldday-sunday, Figma, Fitlad8, Flangiel, Flewis, Florentino floro, Fluffybun, Flyguy649, Fodo96, Fonzy, France3470, Fratrep, Freakofnurture, Freddyd945, Freecat, FreplySpang, Freqsh0, Frodo Muijzer, Frymaster, GTBacchus, Gabbe, Gadfium, Gail, Gaius Cornelius, Garion96, Gary2863, Gazman 1874, Gbleem, Gdo01, Generalkornrow, George The Dragon, George100, Gggh, Gilliam, Glenn, Gnusmas, Gogo Dodo, Gopher292, GraemeHR, GraemeL, Grunty Thraveswain, Guilingkwek, Gurch, Gurry, GustavoBarbieri, Gökhan, H8erade, Hadal, Haham hanuka, Hairy Dude, Hall Monitor, Hallenrm, HamburgerRadio, Handy Pack, Hasek is the best, Hellbus, Henryodell, Herbee, Heron, Hersfold tool account, HexaChord, Heyholetsgoitstimeformmyshow, HiDrNick, Hintswen, Holybarbarian125, Hongooi, Honguy86, Htra0497, Huaiwei, Hurricane111, Husond, Hut 8.5, Hydrogen Iodide, IZAK, IceCreamAntisocial, Iced Kola, Icseaturtles, Ihcoyc, Ilario, Im gonna mock u'z, Intelligentsium, InvaderJim42, Iothiania, Iridescent, Irishguy, Isamedina, Ixfd64, J.delanoy, J.smith, JDoorjam, JRHorse, JVinocur, JYi, JackSparrow Ninja, Jackaranga, Jackol, Jackrace, Javert, JavierMC, Jdrewitt, Jebba, Jeff G., Jeffrey O. Gustafson, Jehnidiah, Jellotine, Jeltz, JensNeu, Jerry Zhang, Jezhotwells, Jfdwolff, Jh12, Jiddisch, Jigesh, JinJian, JingleBells, Jjkusaf, Jni, Joehall45, Joel.delima, Johnakabean, JohnnyCashIsNotDead, Johnpseudo, Johnrpenner, Johser001, Jojhutton, Jojojofook, Jonsilva, Jorvik, Jose77, Josh3580, JoshuaZ, Jossi, Jovianeye, Joyous!, Jredmond, Julesd, Juliancolton, Junk Jungle, Jusdafax, Jóna Þórunn, K.Nevelsteen, KJS77, KPH2293, Kablammo, Kaio393, Kaisershatner, Kakofonous, Kariteh, Katieh5584, Keegan, Keilana, Kierano, Kigoe, Kikos, Kilfoylea, Kim Bruning, Kimyu12, King of Hearts, Kingpin13, Kipala, Kirrages, Kitch, Kmccoy, KnightRider, Knotnic, Kochipoik, Kolindigo, Korath, Kozuch, Kpjas, Kraftlos, Kralizec!, Krash, Krich, Kristen Eriksen, Krun, Kubigula, Kudret abi, Kurt Shaped Box, Kuru, KyNephi, Kyoko, LAAFan, Lacrimosus, Laladu1982, Laurens-af, Lbeben, LeaveSleaves, Leslie Mateus, Leuko, Lexor, LiDaobing, Lightmouse, LinDrug, Linas, Littlewood, Localzhee, Lokicarbis, Lommer, Lordmetroid, Lowellian, Lozzalicious, Lradrama, Lreynol, LtPowers, Luk, Luna Santin, Luqui, MCR.rox.my.world, MER-C, MONGO, MZMcBride, Mac Davis, Macboff, Macintosh User, Maddie!, Madhav, Madhero88, MagneticFlux, Magnus Manske, Majorly, MamaGeek, Man vyi, Manegro, Mani1, Manny gunz, Mantavani, Mapetite526, Marcika, Marcoscramer, Marek69, Mario Luigi, Martin451, Martinwilke1980, Maruti nandan, Masamage, Master1ryan, Matijap, Matt Deres, MattieTK, Mav, Max Naylor, MaxSem, Maximaximax, McDogm, Mdpickle, Me123456789, Medrise, Meeples, Mefanch, Memethor, Menchi, Mendaliv, Mentifisto, MercuryBlue, Merovingian, Mgiganteus1, Mgmei, Mia2009, Michael93555, MightyWarrior, Mikael Häggström, Mikcohen, Mike Rosoft, Mike6271, Mikker, Minghong, Miniyazz, Miquonranger03, MisterKS, Montrealais, Moogle001, Moyogo, Mpt, MrDolomite, MrFish, Mtd2006, MuZemike, Murgatroyd, Myanw, Mygerardromance, Mysid, Møk3, NCurse, NKSCF, Nakon, Naohiro19, Nathan J. Hamilton, NawlinWiki, Nburden, Nemu, Neostarbuck, Nephron, Nescio, Neurolysis, Neutrality, NewEnglandYankee, Newsaholic, Nichalp, Nick, NickBush24, NickGorton, Nicke L, Nidhal79, Night Gyr, Nigosh, Nimbusania, Ninjadalton, Nivix, Nlu, No Guru, Nobuya, Notinasnaid, Nsaa, Nssbm117, NuclearWarfare, Numbo3, Nuno Tavares, Nunquam Dormio, Nuttycoconut, O, ONUnicorn, Obli, Od22, Oda Mari, Oden, OldakQuill, Ollem, Oneiros, Orderud, OttoMäkelä, Ouishoebean, Owen, Owned45, Oxymoron83, PFHLai, PS2pcGAMER, PTSE, Paaskynen, Pablomartinez, PacmanMasterisback, Paigntonuk, Palica, Parthian Scribe, Parvazbato59, Patrick, PatrikR, Patxi lurra, Pavz01, Pax85, Pbiimgp, Pepsidrinka, Peripitus, PeruvianIlama, Peteparker, Peter, Philip Trueman, PhilipMW, Phoenix-forgotten, Pip2andahalf, Pisean282, Plm209, Pmaguire, Pmcalduff, Preston47, PrestonH, Prodego, Proofreader77, Propeng, Pshahmumbai, Psymier, Puchiko, Purgatory Fubar, Purplepalsss, Pyrrhus16, Quantpole, Quatermass, Queen Ele 111, Quinsareth, Qwertyu868, R'n'B, RUL3R, RainbowOfLight, Raisesdead, Ramonesnumer1fan, RaseaC, Raudys, Raven in Orbit, RayAYang, Raysacks, Rcej, Rdsmith4, Rdysn5, Red Thunder, RedHillian, Renato Caniatti, Rettetast, RexNL, Rgoodermote, RhiannonAmelie, Rhysoverton, Riana, Rich Farmbrough, RichardF, Richardcavell, Rlevse, Rob Lindsey, Rocastelo, Rodsan18, Roisinxx, Ronhjones, Ronz, Rrburke, Rror, Rsheridan6, S3000, SCOOTTR666, SJP, SMC, SV Resolution, SWAdair, Sam sam sam88, Samatarou, Samir, Samsara, Samw, Satori Son, SchfiftyThree, SchuminWeb, Scottalter, Seb az86556, Sedmic, Semperf, Senator Palpatine, Sephiroth BCR, Sfdan, Shadowjams, Shanes, Shantavira, Sheitan, Shereth, Shohag, Shoy, Silverhand, Silverleaftree, Simile, SimonMayer, Sintaku, Sionus, Sir Nicholas de Mimsy-Porpington, Sir Vicious, Sjakkalle, Skarebo, Skunkboy74, SkyWalker, Slackerboss, Smalljim, Smitty5555555555, Snowmanradio, SoSaysChappy, Socrates SLB KA, Sodium, Soliloquial, Solitude, SomeStranger, Someguy1221, Sonhyangel, Sonjaaa, Soosed, SpaceFlight89, SpeedyGonsales, SpiderJon, Spitfire, Springnuts, Squirepants101, Sr. farts alot, Stanwhit607, StaticGull, StaticSignals, StaticVision, Stephenb, Stevegray, Stevenfruitsmaak, Stifynsemons, Stink weasel, Strait, Stroppolo, Suffusion of Yellow, Suicidalhamster, SuperHamster, SuperTycoon, Supten, Swaq, Swpb, Sylis9, Synchronism, Syndicate, Syvanen, THEN WHO WAS PHONE?, TShilo12, Talkie tim, Tarret, TastyPoutine, Tavakoli543, Tech77jp, Techman224, Technick29, Template namespace initialisation script, Tempodivalse, TeslaMaster, Tevus, Tgv8925, ThaddeusB, The Anome, The Mad Echidna, The Rambling Man, The Red, The Thing That Should Not Be, The ever man, TheCatalyst31, TheSuave, Thejerm, Thelb4, Theodore Kloba, Thingg, Think outside the box, Thisisajm, Thomas.Nelson05, Thumperward, Thunderboltz, Tide rolls, TigerShark, Tim1988, Timir2, Tiptoety, Tlesher, Tmaguild, Todd Vierling, Tohd8BohaithuGh1, Tom.k, Tonoe84, Tonymaric, Travelbird, Tregoweth, Tresiden, Trevor MacInnis, Tristanb, TubularWorld, Uannis, Ugen64, Uirauna, Unschool, User27091, Utcursch, VFDA, VI, Vanka5, Vatic7, Vegetable4, Verbal, Versageek, Versus22, Violetriga, Vipinhari, Vishnu2011, Viton, Voltron, W746ehj, WLU, WODUP, Waggers, Walid Ashinehgar, Wallaeyozaah, Wapcaplet, Wayne, Weeliljimmy, Wenli, WereSpielChequers, Who, Why Not A Duck, Wiki Super Guardian, Wiki alf, Wiki0709, Wikieditor94, WikieditorOOX, WikipedianMarlith, William Avery, Williammande, Willking1979, Wilstrup, Wimt, Wjfox2005, Wol1i3, Wolfrock, Wompa99, Woohookitty, Worldchanger816, Wouterstomp, Wperdue, Wrad, Writerite, Wshun, Wtmitchell, X0cbabii0x, X201, Xabi17, Xanzzibar, Xcentaur, Xiahou, Xris0, Yamamoto Ichiro, Yekrats, Yomangani, Zantolak, Zazou, ZimZalaBim, Zinneke, Zippo12341234, Zurishaddai, Zvika, Zzuuzz, 2120 anonymous edits

Paracetamol *Source*: http://en.wikipedia.org/w/index.php?oldid=339792645 *Contributors*: 280762nJ, ABCD, ASH1977LAW, Admrboltz, Ageo020, Ahoerstemeier, Ajarmstrong, Akofalvi, Al001, Alansohn, AlbertHall, Alex.tan, Alexwcovington, Alison, Alnokta, AmadeoV, Andreas Rejbrand, Andrew73, Andries, Aneeshjoseph1091, Annmarena, Anrie, Ansett, Antilived, Arcadian, Arjun G. Menon, Assassin3577, AssetBurned, Astavats, Audayan, AxelBoldt, Axl, BATE Borisov, Badgettrg, Baldur, BalthCat, Bardak, Bcorr, Bd1515, Beetstra, Ben.c.roberts, Bender235, Benjah-bmm27, Bezoomy, Bilz0r, Bk0, Blake-, Blue520, Bobet, Booksworm, BorgHunter, BorgQueen, Borgx, Brighterorange, Bryan Derksen, Bsimmons666, Buck Mulligan, BurtonH0123, C6541, Calvero JP, Capricorn42, Casforty, Caspian, Ccroberts, Cdc, Centrx, Chameleon, Chemistbrian, Chensiyuan, Chewie, Cholerashot, Christianpiga, Chrysaor, Citysave, Ck lostsword, CnorthMSU, Coelomic, Colonel Warden, Coollettuce, CrazyChemGuy, Cryonic, Cybercobra, Cú Faoil, DGtal, DHeyward, DMacks, DVirus101, Dakoman, Dan100, DanMatan, Dancraggs, Darthelmo, David Gerard, David.Throop, Davidruben, Deepakvvs, Delpino, DementedPinoy, Derek.cashman, Diberri, Donreed, Drkijewel, Drphilharmonic, Drseudo, Dthomsen8, E kwan, Ed Fitzgerald, Edgar181, Editor182, Edward, EeZbub, Eequor, Egpetersen, Ehn, El C, El3ctr0nika, Eleassar, Eleigh33, Ellywa, Enochlau, Enviroboy, Erich gasboy, Eubulides, Evil saltine, Exabyte, Fairychild, Falcon8765, Filll, Flaskis, FlyHigh, Frappyjohn, Freak0201, Fredrik, Freerick, Frogplate2001, Fuzbaby, Fuzzform, Fvasconcellos, G-Man, Gaius Cornelius, Galaxiaad, Galoubet, Garydh, Gaviidae, Gentgeen, Geoffrey.landis, Gmaxwell, GraemeL, Graingert, GregorB, Grendelkhan, Grimhim, Groodle, GrooveDog, Gunny01, Gustavb, Guy Peters, Hadal, Hahaha123321, Haham hanuka, Hairy Dude, Harthacnut, Hd, Hede2000, HedgeHog, Helixblue, Heshamdiab116, Hopiakuta, HoserHead, Hu12, IRP, IlyaV, Indon, InitHello, InsufficientData, Iorsh, Isaachsieh, Ixfd64, J04n, JForget, JWSchmidt, James.Spudeman, Jamoche, Jcairns123, Jcravino, JeLuF, Jeeves, Jeff G., JeffieFreedom, Jeffrey Mall, Jfdwolff, Jilplo Haggins, Jim Sowers, Jim.Liu, Jklsc, Jmh649, Joel Mc, Johan Lont, John, John Nevard, Johner, Johnuniq, Josh Cherry, Joshuajohnlee, Joy, Juliancolton, Jwestbrook, Jwk, Kajerm, KaragouniS, Karora, Kaustav bose, Kcr, Kd4ttc, Ke4roh, Kevin Murray, Kg6cvv, KirrVlad, Kosebamse, Kozuch, Kp ruddin, Kpjas, Ksheka, Kukulod, Kwamikagami, Kyoko, Lcgarcia, Learo05, Lethaniol, Lexor, Lightmouse, Ligulem, Lokidma, LonelyMarble, Loom91, Louis, Lstanley, Luna Santin, MCB, MER-C, Maccoinnich, Macrakis, MagneticFlux, Malerin, Malo, Mani1, Maralia, Marek69, Mark, Mark ong, MarkGallagher, Markhoney, Marknew, Markthemac, MastCell, Matt Crypto, Matt83au, MatthewJS, Mattworld, Mav, MaxEnt, MaxPont, Maximus Rex, Mayet666, Mazca, Mccready, Medos2, Mernen, Metalhead94, Michael Hardy, Mikr18, Minesweeper, MistyHora, Mitch Ames, Mjb, Mohammad Qasim, Molkhal, Mollwollfumble, Montrealais, Moulder, Mr Bungle, Mr. Billion, Mullet, Myredroom, Naddy, Nahum Reduta, Navicular, Nephron, Neurolysis, Nigelloring, Nldhiep, Notheruser, Nsevs, Nunh-huh, OMGsplosion, OMaj, Oblivious, Officiallyover, Ohnoitsjamie, Oli b, Omicronpersei8, Oxymoron83, Pacula, Parksdh, Patxi lurra, Paul gene, Pavlemocilac, Perspeculum, PeteThePill, Peter Greenwell, Pharmaboy07, Pharmakon logy, Phasmatisnox, Philbert2.71828, Physchim62, Pikiwyn, Pne, PoiZaN, Pol098, Pollinator, Prithason, Prodego, Protox, Pseudomonas, Purple, Pvosta, Quadell, Ququ, R, RG2, Radical Mallard, Raeky, Ral315, Raul654, Raven4x4x, Razorflame, RedWolf, Remember, RexNL, Rhombus, Rich Farmbrough, Richard D. LeCour, Rifleman 82, RingMaruf, Rjwilmsi, Rlcantwell, Rmhermen, RobertG, Rodhullandemu, Ronhjones, Rosenknospe, RossPatterson, Rrburke, SP-KP, SRE.K.A.L.24, Salvadorjo, Sambridger, Samuel Pepys, SandyGeorgia, Sanfranman59, Sapphic, Sarangk2005, Sayeth, Sceptre, Scott Wilson, Scray, Sekio, Senseiwa, Sesmith, Seven of Nine, Shadowjams, ShaunES, Shinhan, Shipondu, Sikkema, Simicich, SimonP, Simonsez4242, SineWave, Sir Drance, Siroxo, Skier Dude, SmilingBoy, Snappyfool, Snickerdo, Sonett72, Sonjaaa, Soundoftoday, Spencer195, Spinningobo, Starrycutie, Stay cool, Stevenfruitsmaak, Stmrlbs, Stone, Stugen, Stylese, Subclavian, Sunborn, Sunriseshell, Supparluca, Surachit, Sushiflinger, Susurrus, Swatjester, Synergy, T0rek, Tangent747, Tarquin, Taxman, Techelf, Tempodivalse, The Anome, The Rambling Man, The Right Honourable, TheMandarin, ThePianoMan, Thebonefabric, Thekaekara99, Thomas fischer, Thoric, ThreeBlindMice, Tide rolls, TimVickers, Timos55, Tjmayerinsf, Tkynerd, Tlesher, Tomaxer, Tonigonenstein, Treisijs, TreyHarris, Tristanb, Trlkly, Trungdung Mai, Tryxiex, Tut akhen amon, Tybalt01, Ultramarine, Una Smith, Urbanbicyclist, Uthbrian, V8rik, Variant, Varlaam, Veesicle, Vendettax, Vetedit1982, Vicki Rosenzweig, VigilancePrime, Vinney, Voidxor, Wadems, Walkerma, Walor, WhatamIdoing, Where next Columbus?, Whereizben, Wikibofh, Williadb, William mcfadden, WillowW, Wimvandorst, Woohookitty, Wouterstomp, Wtmitchell, Wyatt915, X1987x, Xasodfuih, XxPantherNovaXx, Zandperl, Zaphraud, ZayZayEM, Zedla, Zephyris, [212], 689 anonymous edits

Ibuprofen *Source*: http://en.wikipedia.org/w/index.php?oldid=340141058 *Contributors*: A2Kafir, Adam McMaster, Afasmit, Ahoerstemeier, Aka, Aldis90, Alethiophile, AlexanderWinston, Ali@gwc.org.uk, Almazi, Anastrophe, Ank329, Ansett, Anypodetos, Arcadian, ArglebargleIV, Ashley Pomeroy, Audry2, Axlq, Ayeroxor, B-D, Babbage, Beetstra, Bekuletz, Beland, Ben Arnold, Bender235, Benjah-bmm27, Bettia, Bezapt, Bhadani, BiggKwell, Blinq, Blukens, Bmramon, Bobo192, Bogwhistle, Brianga, Brighterorange, Brokenchairs, Bryan Derksen, Bugzptr, Bull Winkus, CERminator, Cacycle, CalebNoble, Can't sleep, clown will eat me, Carloseduardo, Carolfrog, Casforty, Chameleon, Charles Matthews, Chem-awb, ChildOfLore, Chris01720, Cp111, CrazyChemGuy, Crazycomputers, Cssiitcic, Custardninja, Cybercobra, Dan100, DanMS, Dancraggs, DarkFalls, Dasani, Davemc50, Davidruben, Dbutler1986, Dchristle, Derek.cashman, Derek6193, Discospinster, DocWatson42, Donmike10, Dosai, Dr R Bowri, Drini, Drumguy8800, Duncan.france, Dylar, Dyslexik, E0steven, ERcheck, Ed Fitzgerald, Eequor, Efajo, Eionm, Eleassar, Emperorbma, Epbr123, Eras-mus, Eric Kvaalen, Errol tash, Esperant, Etatoby, EvilStorm, Facts707, Fail, Fconaway, Fieldday-sunday, Flyguy649, Freestyle-69, Fuzzform, Fvasconcellos, GOD ACRONYM, Galaxiaad, Gaviidae, GeeCee, Geographer, Gilgamesh, Giulit, GraemeL, GreenReaper, Gregfitzy, Ground Zero, Gsingh, Gubernator, Gurch, Gutzmer, Gwernol, Haikupoet, Halim289, Hao2lian, Harbinary, HedgeHog, Heron, Hlinz, Hydrargyrum, IByte, IMSoP, Iliko, ImperfectlyInformed, Iridescent, J.delanoy, J04n, JFreeman, Jak123,

Article Sources and Contributors

Jakezing, JamieS93, Javsav, Jaxl, Jcmaco, Jeremy68, Jerzy, Jfdwolff, Jklin, John, Johnnypuffs, Josh3580, Jossi, Joy, Jweiss11, Jū, K.d.stauffer, K33l0r, Kajmal, Katari Devi, Katnap01, Kbh3rd, Keppa, Kilbad, King of Hearts, Kjbaldio, KnightRider, Kpjas, Kwamikagami, La goutte de pluie, Latka, Law Lord, Lengman inna dis, LonelyMarble, MJStewart84, Macrakis, Manuella13, Marek69, Marx1326, MasterOfPuppets, Mav, Maxamegalon2000, McGeddon, Messymedic, Miguel Andrade, Mike Segal, Mmxx, Moa3333, Moriori, Morwen, Mr Bungle, MrDarcy, Mstroeck, Muczachan, Mykhal, Neurolysis, Nikka319, Nono64, Nstott, Orangemarlin, P-kun80, PDH, Pabouk, Palamides, Patkica, Paul Gard, Paxsimius, Pd THOR, PeteThePill, Ph.eyes, Philip Trueman, Physicistjedi, Piggggu, Plantsurfer, Pne, Pomzazed, Prisonblues, Prolog, Psiphiorg, Psm, QuentinBurley, Ragesoss, RandomStringOfCharacters, Ravik, Rbmoore, Rboatright, RebootEDC, Rebroad, Rees11, Retroid, Rich Farmbrough, Rifleman 82, Rjwilmsi, Robert Merkel, Rolypolyman, RonDivine, Runt, SP-KP, ST47, Sailormd, Saku kodo, Sango123, Santiago Roza (Kq), Schneelocke, Scientus, Sean Whitton, Sean22190, Septegram, Shotmenot, Shoy, SimonP, Slash, Slipdrive44, Snori, SoWhy, St3vo, Starisaac, Stone, Subversive, Suffusion of Yellow, SupaStarGirl, Superm401, Sushiflinger, Swedan, SwedishPsycho, T0rek, Tannerhelland, Tarndanya, TastyPoutine, Tchalvak, Techelf, Teutonic Tamer, The Right Honourable, The Thing That Should Not Be, TheMandarin, Thecurran, Thedjatclubrock, Thomprod, Tim Q. Wells, Tim bates, Tins128, Tofy792000, Toh, Ugen64, Ugha, Uthbrian, Vantey, Virgo82, WLU, WikiLaurent, Wikipedia is Nazism, Wildcat156, Williadh, Willson50, Wolfkeeper, X!, Xabian40409, Xioxox, Yosefxp, Z-m-k, ZBAUGH, Zulaica, Александър, مرح دماغ عضلي.24, طبال يلع خرسا, 612 anonymous edits

Myocardial infarction Source: http://en.wikipedia.org/w/index.php?oldid=339880650 Contributors: *drew, A Man In Black, AED, AThing, Acegikmo1, Acerperi, Acroterion, Adambiswanger1, AdjustShift, Adriatikus, Ageekgal, Ahoerstemeier, Aiman abmajid, Alanames, Aleenf1, Alex Golub, Alex.tan, AlexBriggs13, AliveFreeHappy, Alphachimp, AnOddName, Andre Engels, Andres, AndrewHowse, Andrewjlockley, Andrewjuren, Andy M. Wang, Angela, Anna Lincoln, Antandrus, Apollo the Archer, Arcadian, ArmadilloFromHell, Aswang, Atlant, Avono, AxelBoldt, Axl, AySz88, Banaticus, Barek, BarkingFish, Barticus88, Bbain, Bdesham, Beetstra, Beland, BenM, Benabik, Benbest, Berean Hunter, Bezapt, Bigboi3, Billfincle, Binduka, Bjackson35, Bleiglass, Blindman shady, Bluerasberry, BobKawanaka, Boback, Bobet, Bobo192, Brianga, Brighterorange, Brockert, Brossow, Brouhardr, Bwrs, C Craig Marshall, C+C, COOTBALLIN, Camden7, Can't sleep, clown will eat me, Capricorn42, Cardioresearch, Catgut, Cdang, Celithemis, Chris Sunderland, Chris the speller, Chrysaor, Cmgibson, Conort10lulz, Cryforhelp, Ctande, Cybercobra, D Dinneen, D00mj, DHN, DOCtraind, Da monster under your bed, DagnyB, Danjeffers, DariaNoelle, Darth Panda, Darwinek, Davidruben, Dawn Bard, Deepbluevibes, Dekisugi, Deli nk, Delldot, DenisDiderot, DerHexer, Det3574, Diberri, DimaDorfman, Discospinster, Displaced, Dlodge, Dlohcierekim, Doctorrobert, Dr.Golovenko, Dr.shivani jaiwal, Drchazz, Dreadstar, Drini, Drru0999, Drslyguy, DubaiTerminator, Dungodung, Dust Filter, Echojahra, Eclectic hippie, Edonald, Edwin, El C, Elizabeyth, Elronxenu, Emperorbma, Enviroboy, Ephr123, Everyking, Evfc8, Excirial, Exor674, Facts707, Ferdy1125, Fieldday-sunday, Fig25, Finlay McWalter, Firsfron, Fledgeling, Florentino floro, Flyguy649, FocalPoint, Foot1647, Foszto, Freshbakedpie, Fuckingeveryone, Fuzheado, Fvasconcellos, Gail, Gaius Cornelius, Gak, Galactor213, Gassy999, Ggogler, Ghostal, Giftlite, Gilliam, Gimlifilmfestival, Glenlarson, Gnusmas, Gogo Dodo, Graemel., Gregoing, Gtdp, Guthrie, Gwernol, H, H Padleckas, Hapsiainen, Harryboyles, Hephaestos, Heroeswithmetaphors, Hfcom, Hhhhnnnngggggggg, Hickorybark, Horsten, Horstie, Hraefen, Hu12, Husond, I'm not giving my name to a machine, II MusLiM HyBRiD II, Iassaiias, Icairns, Icarus, IdahoEv, Impala2009, Ipsingh, Isnow, ItsWoody, J Di, J.delanoy, JVinocur, Jack Daw, Jacoplane, Jakechan, JamesAM, JanEngel, Jared999, Jclemens, Jevav, Jezmck, Jfdwolff, Jhfireboy, Jhon2deer, Jklak, Jmh649, JodyB, Johan1298, John24601, Johnpseudo, Johnuniq, Joseaperez, Julesd, Jwh335, Jóna Pórunn, K keysha, Kaal, Kaobear, Karada, Karl-Henner, Kartano, Kayag, Kd4tte, Keilana, Kemiv, KerryB, Kestrel452, Kirtilad20, Kitch, Kpjas, Krellis, Ksheka, Kylescott27, Kyoko, Larth Rasnal, Leon7, Leungchuenyan, Librarian255, Lightmouse, Lights, Ligulem, Litanss, Lmaltier, Lmuenchen, Lorenjens, Luk, Lyrl, M0rt, MAlvis, MER-C, Macy, Mandarax, Manojmishra5, Mark.murphy, MarsRover, Martpol, MastCell, Materialscientist, Mav, Maximus Rex, Mayfly may fly, Mayooranathan, Mdanciu, Medic, Medrise, Melchoir, Meldor, Menchi, Meno25, Mentifisto, Meske, Mikael Häggström, Mike2vil, Mike71, Mindmatrix, Mintleaf, Mistercollege, Modulatum, Montrealais, MoodyGroove, Moonriddengirl, MrFish, MrRadioGuy, Mygerardromance, N5iln, NCurse, Narge, Natl1, NawlinWiki, Ncurrier, Neil916, Nephron, Newestscientist, Newyorkbrad, Nihiltres, Nmg20, Nopetro, Notinasnaid, Nposs, Nscheffey, Nunh-huh, Nuprin, Nuzz604, OBILI, Ohnoitsjamie, Oliver202, Onco p53, Operon-wiki, Orangemarlin, Orangeroof, Ouroboros0427, Oxymoron83, PGWG, Panterka, ParaGreen13, Patxi lurra, Pb30, Pebene, Peteforsyth, Peter Farago, Peter Gheeraert, Philip Trueman, Philopp, Pilarian, Pisces56, Pproctor, Prashanthns, PrestonH, Pritt tipu, Quadell, Qutezuce, Qwfp, RDBrown, RJ Petry, RajeevA, Rajrajmarley, Rantira, Raquel Baranow, Rasmus Faber, Ravik, Red Act, Redhookesb, Renamed user 1253, Renato Caniatti, RexNL, Rich Farmbrough, RichardSocher, Richardcavell, RickK, Rjwilmsi, Rmrfstar, RobLa, Roberta F., Ronark, Ruhrjung, Ryan-McCulloch, SANITYISFORTHEWEAK, SEWilco, Sam Blacketer, Sangak, Sanguinity, Savorie, Sbbcsb, Scarian, Scope2776, Scwlong, Search4Lancer, Serrano, Sherm8th, Shortdistancerunner, Shze, Silassewell, SiobhanHansa, Sir Fastolfe, Sir Nicholas de Mimsy-Porpington, SirGrant, Sirishapingali1, Snowmanradio, Solaman12, Someone else, SpaceFlight89, Spencer, Spiff666, Spongefrog, Spsycher, Staffwaterboy, Stanislav87, Starry.dreams, Stevenfruitsmaak, Stevertigo, Stwalkerster, Sunidesus, Swizzlez, Syaifulshah, TUF-KAT, Tallasse, Tannim101, Taopman, Tdcmfan11, Techelf, Teridius, The Rambling Man, The Thing That Should Not Be, Thelanton, TheTito, Thingg, Tide rolls, TimVickers, Tivedshambo, Tom Ketchum, Tomaxer, Tombyt55, Tomfarvour, Tristanb, Tutmosis, Tyrasibion, UP3, Ukexpat, Ultra two, Unclfester, Unitycenter, Useight, User F203, Useropsranger, Uthbrian, VFDA, Vadkins100, Vaultdoor, Versus22, Viskonsas, Vsmith, Vuvar1, WLU, Waster, Wawot1, Wiki alf, Wikieditor06, Williamblack444, Willtron, Wouterstomp, Xaosflux, Xiahou, Yasitha2, Yms, ZOOMD, Zephalis, Zigger, Zisimos, Zntrip, Александър, 801 anonymous edits

Image Sources, Licenses and Contributors

File:Verkalkte aneurysmatische Coronarien.jpg *Source*: http://en.wikipedia.org/w/index.php?title=File:Verkalkte_aneurysmatische_Coronarien.jpg *License*: Public Domain *Contributors*: Original uploader was Wkmatzek at de.wikipedia (Original text : wkmatzek)

Image:KAWASAKI1.jpg *Source*: http://en.wikipedia.org/w/index.php?title=File:KAWASAKI1.jpg *License*: Public Domain *Contributors*: User:Dra marina

Image:Skin.jpg *Source*: http://en.wikipedia.org/w/index.php?title=File:Skin.jpg *License*: Public Domain *Contributors*: Denniss, John Biancato, Lennert B, Lipothymia, NikNaks93, 1 anonymous edits

Image:Sa-rhino-skin.jpg *Source*: http://en.wikipedia.org/w/index.php?title=File:Sa-rhino-skin.jpg *License*: GNU Free Documentation License *Contributors*: User:Sanjay ach

Image:HautFingerspitzeOCT nonanimated.gif *Source*: http://en.wikipedia.org/w/index.php?title=File:HautFingerspitzeOCT_nonanimated.gif *License*: Creative Commons Attribution-Sharealike 2.0 *Contributors*: User:Wikid77

Image:Gray942.png *Source*: http://en.wikipedia.org/w/index.php?title=File:Gray942.png *License*: unknown *Contributors*: Arcadian, Magnus Manske, Origamiemensch

Image:Gray940.png *Source*: http://en.wikipedia.org/w/index.php?title=File:Gray940.png *License*: unknown *Contributors*: Arcadian, Magnus Manske, Origamiemensch

Image:Ens.png *Source*: http://en.wikipedia.org/w/index.php?title=File:Ens.png *License*: GNU Free Documentation License *Contributors*: Cayte, SoCalSuperEagle, 1 anonymous edits

Image:Gray1033.png *Source*: http://en.wikipedia.org/w/index.php?title=File:Gray1033.png *License*: unknown *Contributors*: Arcadian, Magnus Manske, Origamiemensch

Image:Illu ureters wall.jpg *Source*: http://en.wikipedia.org/w/index.php?title=File:Illu_ureters_wall.jpg *License*: Public Domain *Contributors*: Arcadian

Image:Gray1053.png *Source*: http://en.wikipedia.org/w/index.php?title=File:Gray1053.png *License*: unknown *Contributors*: Arcadian, DO11.10, Haabet, Magnus Manske, Origamiemensch

Image:Gut wall.svg *Source*: http://en.wikipedia.org/w/index.php?title=File:Gut_wall.svg *License*: Creative Commons Attribution 3.0 *Contributors*: Original uploader was Auawise at en.wikipedia (Original text : Auaʃ Wise (Operibus anteire))

Image:Illu lymph node structure.png *Source*: http://en.wikipedia.org/w/index.php?title=File:Illu_lymph_node_structure.png *License*: Public Domain *Contributors*: SEER

Image:Schematic of lymph node showing lymph sinuses.svg *Source*: http://en.wikipedia.org/w/index.php?title=File:Schematic_of_lymph_node_showing_lymph_sinuses.svg *License*: Public Domain *Contributors*: User:KC Panchal

Image:Lymph node regions.jpg *Source*: http://en.wikipedia.org/w/index.php?title=File:Lymph_node_regions.jpg *License*: Public Domain *Contributors*: http://training.seer.cancer.gov/ss_module08_lymph_leuk/lymph_unit02_sec02_reg_lns.html

Image:Crc met to node1.jpg *Source*: http://en.wikipedia.org/w/index.php?title=File:Crc_met_to_node1.jpg *License*: GNU Free Documentation License *Contributors*: User:Nephron

Image:Illu lymphatic system.jpg *Source*: http://en.wikipedia.org/w/index.php?title=File:Illu_lymphatic_system.jpg *License*: Public Domain *Contributors*: Arcadian, AtonX, 3 anonymous edits

Image:Lymphatic system.png *Source*: http://en.wikipedia.org/w/index.php?title=File:Lymphatic_system.png *License*: Public Domain *Contributors*: NIH

Image:Gray597.png *Source*: http://en.wikipedia.org/w/index.php?title=File:Gray597.png *License*: Public Domain *Contributors*: Arcadian

Image:Gray606.png *Source*: http://en.wikipedia.org/w/index.php?title=File:Gray606.png *License*: Public Domain *Contributors*: Arcadian

Image:Gray607.png *Source*: http://en.wikipedia.org/w/index.php?title=File:Gray607.png *License*: Public Domain *Contributors*: Arcadian

Image:Gray1074.png *Source*: http://en.wikipedia.org/w/index.php?title=File:Gray1074.png *License*: unknown *Contributors*: Arcadian, Magnus Manske, Origamiemensch

Image:Gray1082.png *Source*: http://en.wikipedia.org/w/index.php?title=File:Gray1082.png *License*: unknown *Contributors*: Arcadian, Origamiemensch

Image:Lymphknoten (Schwein).jpg *Source*: http://en.wikipedia.org/w/index.php?title=File:Lymphknoten_(Schwein).jpg *License*: Creative Commons Attribution-Sharealike 2.0 *Contributors*: GleibergOriginal uploader was Gleiberg at de.wikipedia

Image:Circulatory System en.svg *Source*: http://en.wikipedia.org/w/index.php?title=File:Circulatory_System_en.svg *License*: Public Domain *Contributors*: User:LadyofHats

File:Drkawasaki.jpg *Source*: http://en.wikipedia.org/w/index.php?title=File:Drkawasaki.jpg *License*: Public Domain *Contributors*: Dr. Rae Yeung

Image:heart.jpg *Source*: http://en.wikipedia.org/w/index.php?title=File:Heart.jpg *License*: Creative Commons Attribution-Sharealike 2.5 *Contributors*: Heikenwaelder Hugo, heikenwaelder@aon.at, www.heikenwaelder.at

Image:EHR-BBII.jpg *Source*: http://en.wikipedia.org/w/index.php?title=File:EHR-BBII.jpg *License*: unknown *Contributors*: Bek the Conqueror, Brighterorange, Bsadowski1, Dibern, DuBose, MithrandirMage, Vinsfan368, 4 anonymous edits

Image:Humhrt2.jpg *Source*: http://en.wikipedia.org/w/index.php?title=File:Humhrt2.jpg *License*: unknown *Contributors*: User:Ewen

Image:Surface anatomy of the heart.png *Source*: http://en.wikipedia.org/w/index.php?title=File:Surface_anatomy_of_the_heart.png *License*: Public Domain *Contributors*: Mikael Häggström

Image:Gunshot heart.jpg *Source*: http://en.wikipedia.org/w/index.php?title=File:Gunshot_heart.jpg *License*: Public Domain *Contributors*: National Institutes of Health, Health & Human Services

File:Paracetamol-skeletal.svg *Source*: http://en.wikipedia.org/w/index.php?title=File:Paracetamol-skeletal.svg *License*: Public Domain *Contributors*: Benjah-bmm27

File:Paracetamol-from-xtal-3D-balls.png *Source*: http://en.wikipedia.org/w/index.php?title=File:Paracetamol-from-xtal-3D-balls.png *License*: Public Domain *Contributors*: Ben Mills

Image:Yes check.svg *Source*: http://en.wikipedia.org/w/index.php?title=File:Yes_check.svg *License*: Public Domain *Contributors*: User:Gmaxwell, User:WarX

File:Speaker Icon.svg *Source*: http://en.wikipedia.org/w/index.php?title=File:Speaker_Icon.svg *License*: Public Domain *Contributors*: Blast, G.Hagedorn, Mobius, 2 anonymous edits

Image:Axelrod.jpg *Source*: http://en.wikipedia.org/w/index.php?title=File:Axelrod.jpg *License*: Public Domain *Contributors*: National Institutes of Health

Image:Polar-surface-area.png *Source*: http://en.wikipedia.org/w/index.php?title=File:Polar-surface-area.png *License*: Public Domain *Contributors*: User:Molecool

Image:Synthesis of paracetamol from phenol.png *Source*: http://en.wikipedia.org/w/index.php?title=File:Synthesis_of_paracetamol_from_phenol.png *License*: Public Domain *Contributors*: User:Rifleman 82

Image:Panadol.jpg *Source*: http://en.wikipedia.org/w/index.php?title=File:Panadol.jpg *License*: Public Domain *Contributors*: Editor182

Image:AM404 skel.png *Source*: http://en.wikipedia.org/w/index.php?title=File:AM404_skel.png *License*: Creative Commons Attribution-Sharealike 3.0 *Contributors*: User:Xasodfuih

Image:Anandamide skeletal.svg *Source*: http://en.wikipedia.org/w/index.php?title=File:Anandamide_skeletal.svg *License*: Public Domain *Contributors*: User:Fvasconcellos

Image:Paracetamol metabolism.svg *Source*: http://en.wikipedia.org/w/index.php?title=File:Paracetamol_metabolism.svg *License*: Public Domain *Contributors*: Fvasconcellos

File:Ibuprofen.svg *Source*: http://en.wikipedia.org/w/index.php?title=File:Ibuprofen.svg *License*: Public Domain *Contributors*: User:Harbin

Image:200mg ibuprofen tablets.jpg *Source*: http://en.wikipedia.org/w/index.php?title=File:200mg_ibuprofen_tablets.jpg *License*: Creative Commons Attribution-Sharealike 3.0 *Contributors*: User:Ragesoss

Image:R-ibuprofen-B-2D-skeletal.png *Source*: http://en.wikipedia.org/w/index.php?title=File:R-ibuprofen-B-2D-skeletal.png *License*: Public Domain *Contributors*: User:Benjah-bmm27

Image:S-ibuprofen-A-2D-skeletal.png *Source*: http://en.wikipedia.org/w/index.php?title=File:S-ibuprofen-A-2D-skeletal.png *License*: Public Domain *Contributors*: User:Benjah-bmm27

Image:R-ibuprofen-A-2D-skeletal.png *Source*: http://en.wikipedia.org/w/index.php?title=File:R-ibuprofen-A-2D-skeletal.png *License*: Public Domain *Contributors*: User:Benjah-bmm27

Image:S-ibuprofen-B-2D-skeletal.png *Source*: http://en.wikipedia.org/w/index.php?title=File:S-ibuprofen-B-2D-skeletal.png *License*: Public Domain *Contributors*: User:Benjah-bmm27

Image:Ibuprofen-3D-balls.png *Source*: http://en.wikipedia.org/w/index.php?title=File:Ibuprofen-3D-balls.png *License*: Public Domain *Contributors*: User:Benjah-bmm27

Image:(S)-ibuprofen-3D-balls.png *Source*: http://en.wikipedia.org/w/index.php?title=File:(S)-ibuprofen-3D-balls.png *License*: Public Domain *Contributors*: User:Benjah-bmm27

File:Boots synthesis of ibuprofen.png *Source*: http://en.wikipedia.org/w/index.php?title=File:Boots_synthesis_of_ibuprofen.png *License*: Public Domain *Contributors*: User:Rifleman 82

File:BHC synthesis of ibuprofen.png *Source*: http://en.wikipedia.org/w/index.php?title=File:BHC_synthesis_of_ibuprofen.png *License*: Public Domain *Contributors*: User:Rifleman 82

File:Generic Ipubrofen.JPG *Source*: http://en.wikipedia.org/w/index.php?title=File:Generic_Ipubrofen.JPG *License*: Public Domain *Contributors*: User:Donmike10

File:AMI scheme.png *Source*: http://en.wikipedia.org/w/index.php?title=File:AMI_scheme.png *License*: unknown *Contributors*: User:JHeuser

Image:AMI pain front.png *Source*: http://en.wikipedia.org/w/index.php?title=File:AMI_pain_front.png *License*: GNU Free Documentation License *Contributors*: User:JHeuser

Image:AMI pain back.png *Source*: http://en.wikipedia.org/w/index.php?title=File:AMI_pain_back.png *License*: GNU Free Documentation License *Contributors*: User:JHeuser

Image:Heart attack diagram.png *Source*: http://en.wikipedia.org/w/index.php?title=File:Heart_attack_diagram.png *License*: Public Domain *Contributors*: Cwbm (commons), Kjetil r, The cat, 1 anonymous edits

Image Sources, Licenses and Contributors

Image:12 Lead EKG ST Elevation tracing color coded.jpg *Source*: http://en.wikipedia.org/w/index.php?title=File:12_Lead_EKG_ST_Elevation_tracing_color_coded.jpg *License*: Public Domain *Contributors*: User:Displaced

Image:Ha1.jpg *Source*: http://en.wikipedia.org/w/index.php?title=File:Ha1.jpg *License*: unknown *Contributors*: Dodo

Image:Myocardial infarct emmolition phase histopathology.jpg *Source*: http://en.wikipedia.org/w/index.php?title=File:Myocardial_infarct_emmolition_phase_histopathology.jpg *License*: Public Domain *Contributors*: Alex brollo, Ares.it, Kwz, 4 anonymous edits

Image:MI with contraction bands very high mag.jpg *Source*: http://en.wikipedia.org/w/index.php?title=File:MI_with_contraction_bands_very_high_mag.jpg *License*: GNU Free Documentation License *Contributors*: User:Nephron

Image:Intracoronary thrombus.png *Source*: http://en.wikipedia.org/w/index.php?title=File:Intracoronary_thrombus.png *License*: Creative Commons Attribution-Sharealike 2.5 *Contributors*: Original uploader was Ksheka at en.wikipedia

Image:Coronary artery bypass surgery Image 657B-PH.jpg *Source*: http://en.wikipedia.org/w/index.php?title=File:Coronary_artery_bypass_surgery_Image_657B-PH.jpg *License*: unknown *Contributors*: Original uploader was SeanMack at en.wikipedia

Image:Electrocardiogram of Ventricular Tachycardia.png *Source*: http://en.wikipedia.org/w/index.php?title=File:Electrocardiogram_of_Ventricular_Tachycardia.png *License*: Creative Commons Attribution-Sharealike 2.5 *Contributors*: Original uploader was Ksheka at en.wikipedia

License

Creative Commons Attribution-Share Alike 3.0 Unported
http://creativecommons.org/licenses/by-sa/3.0/

VDM publishing house ltd.

Scientific Publishing House

offers

free of charge publication

of current academic research papers, Bachelor´s Theses, Master's Theses, Dissertations or Scientific Monographs

If you have written a thesis which satisfies high content as well as formal demands, and you are interested in a remunerated publication of your work, please send an e-mail with some initial information about yourself and your work to *info@vdm-publishing-house.com*.

Our editorial office will get in touch with you shortly.

VDM Publishing House Ltd.
Meldrum Court 17.
Beau Bassin
Mauritius
www.vdm-publishing-house.com

GNU Free Documentation License Version 1.2, November 2002 Copyright (C) 2000,2001,2002 Free Software Foundation, Inc. 59 Temple Place, Suite 330, Boston, MA 02111-1307 USA Everyone is permitted to copy and distribute verbatim copies of this license document, but changing it is not allowed.

0. PREAMBLE

The purpose of this License is to make a manual, textbook, or other functional and useful document "free" in the sense of freedom: to assure everyone the effective freedom to copy and redistribute it, with or without modifying it, either commercially or noncommercially. Secondarily, this License preserves for the author and publisher a way to get credit for their work, while not being considered responsible for modifications made by others. This License is a kind of "copyleft", which means that derivative works of the document must themselves be free in the same sense. It complements the GNU General Public License, which is a copyleft license designed for free software. We have designed this License in order to use it for manuals for free software, because free software needs free documentation: a free program should come with manuals providing the same freedoms that the software does. But this License is not limited to software manuals; it can be used for any textual work, regardless of subject matter or whether it is published as a printed book. We recommend this License principally for works whose purpose is instruction or reference.

1. APPLICABILITY AND DEFINITIONS

This License applies to any manual or other work, in any medium, that contains a notice placed by the copyright holder saying it can be distributed under the terms of this License. Such a notice grants a world-wide, royalty-free license, unlimited in duration, to use that work under the conditions stated herein. The "Document", below, refers to any such manual or work. Any member of the public is a licensee, and is addressed as "you". You accept the license if you copy, modify or distribute the work in a way requiring permission under copyright law. A "Modified Version" of the Document means any work containing the Document or a portion of it, either copied verbatim, or with modifications and/or translated into another language. A "Secondary Section" is a named appendix or a front-matter section of the Document that deals exclusively with the relationship of the publishers or authors of the Document to the Document's overall subject (or to related matters) and contains nothing that could fall directly within that overall subject. (Thus, if the Document is in part a textbook of mathematics, a Secondary Section may not explain any mathematics.) The relationship could be a matter of historical connection with the subject or with related matters, or of legal, commercial, philosophical, ethical or political position regarding them. The "Invariant Sections" are certain Secondary Sections whose titles are designated, as being those of Invariant Sections, in the notice that says that the Document is released under this License. If a section does not fit the above definition of Secondary then it is not allowed to be designated as Invariant. The Document may contain zero Invariant Sections. If the Document does not identify any Invariant Sections then there are none. The "Cover Texts" are certain short passages of text that are listed, as Front-Cover Texts or Back-Cover Texts, in the notice that says that the Document is released under this License. A Front-Cover Text may be at most 5 words, and a Back-Cover Text may be at most 25 words. A "Transparent" copy of the Document means a machine-readable copy, represented in a format whose specification is available to the general public, that is suitable for revising the document straightforwardly with generic text editors or (for images composed of pixels) generic paint programs or (for drawings) some widely available drawing editor, and that is suitable for input to text formatters or for automatic translation to a variety of formats suitable for input to text formatters. A copy made in an otherwise Transparent file format whose markup, or absence of markup, has been arranged to thwart or discourage subsequent modification by readers is not Transparent. An image format is not Transparent if used for any substantial amount of text. A copy that is not "Transparent" is called "Opaque". Examples of suitable formats for Transparent copies include plain ASCII without markup, Texinfo input format, LaTeX input format, SGML or XML using a publicly available DTD, and standard-conforming simple HTML, PostScript or PDF designed for human modification. Examples of transparent image formats include PNG, XCF and JPG. Opaque formats include proprietary formats that can be read and edited only by proprietary word processors, SGML or XML for which the DTD and/or processing tools are not generally available, and the machine-generated HTML, PostScript or PDF produced by some word processors for output purposes only. The "Title Page" means, for a printed book, the title page itself, plus such following pages as are needed to hold, legibly, the material this License requires to appear in the title page. For works in formats which do not have any title page as such, "Title Page" means the text near the most prominent appearance of the work's title, preceding the beginning of the body of the text. A section Entitled "XYZ" means a named subunit of the Document whose title either is precisely XYZ or contains XYZ in parentheses following text that translates XYZ in another language. (Here XYZ stands for a specific section name mentioned below, such as "Acknowledgements", "Dedications", "Endorsements", or "History".) To "Preserve the Title" of such a section when you modify the Document means that it remains a section "Entitled XYZ" according to this definition. The Document may include Warranty Disclaimers next to the notice which states that this License applies to the Document. These Warranty Disclaimers are considered to be included by reference in this License, but only as regards disclaiming warranties: any other implication that these Warranty Disclaimers may have is void and has no effect on the meaning of this License.

2. VERBATIM COPYING

You may copy and distribute the Document in any medium, either commercially or noncommercially, provided that this License, the copyright notices, and the license notice saying this License applies to the Document are reproduced in all copies, and that you add no other conditions whatsoever to those of this License. You may not use technical measures to obstruct or control the reading or further copying of the copies you make or distribute. However, you may accept compensation in exchange for copies. If you distribute a large enough number of copies you must also follow the conditions in section 3. You may also lend copies, under the same conditions stated above, and you may publicly display copies.

3. COPYING IN QUANTITY

If you publish printed copies (or copies in media that commonly have printed covers) of the Document, numbering more than 100, and the Document's license notice requires Cover Texts, you must enclose the copies in covers that carry, clearly and legibly, all these Cover Texts: Front-Cover Texts on the front cover, and Back-Cover Texts on the back cover. Both covers must also clearly and legibly identify you as the publisher of these copies. The front cover must present the full title with all words of the title equally prominent and visible. You may add other material on the covers in addition. Copying with changes limited to the covers, as long as they preserve the title of the Document and satisfy these conditions, can be treated as verbatim copying in other respects. If the required texts for either cover are too voluminous to fit legibly, you should put the first ones listed (as many as fit reasonably) on the actual cover, and continue the rest onto adjacent pages. If you publish or distribute Opaque copies of the Document numbering more than 100, you must either include a machine-readable Transparent copy along with each Opaque copy, or state in or with each Opaque copy a computer-network location from which the general network-using public has access to download using public-standard network protocols a complete Transparent copy of the Document, free of added material. If you use the latter option, you must take reasonably prudent steps, when you begin distribution of Opaque copies in quantity, to ensure that this Transparent copy will remain thus accessible at the stated location until at least one year after the last time you distribute an Opaque copy (directly or through your agents or retailers) of that edition to the public. It is requested, but not required, that you contact the authors of the Document well before redistributing any large number of copies, to give them a chance to provide you with an updated version of the Document.

4. MODIFICATIONS

You may copy and distribute a Modified Version of the Document under the conditions of sections 2 and 3 above, provided that you release the Modified Version under precisely this License, with the Modified Version filling the role of the Document, thus licensing distribution and modification of the Modified Version to whoever possesses a copy of it. In addition, you must do these things in the Modified Version: A. Use in the Title Page (and on the covers, if any) a title distinct from that of the Document, and from those of previous versions (which should, if there were any, be listed in the History section of the Document). You may use the same title as a previous version if the original publisher of that version gives permission. B. List on the Title Page, as authors, one or more persons or entities responsible for authorship of the modifications in the Modified Version, together with at least five of the principal authors of the Document (all of its principal authors, if it has fewer than five), unless they release you from this requirement. C. State on the Title page the name of the publisher of the Modified Version, as the publisher. D. Preserve all the copyright notices of the Document. E. Add an appropriate copyright notice for your modifications adjacent to the other copyright notices. F. Include, immediately after the copyright notices, a license notice giving the public permission to use the Modified Version under the terms of this License, in the form shown in the Addendum below. G. Preserve in that license notice the full lists of Invariant Sections and required Cover Texts given in the Document's license notice. H. Include an unaltered copy of this License. I. Preserve the section Entitled "History", Preserve its Title, and add to it an item stating at least the title, year, new authors, and publisher of the Modified Version as given on the Title Page. If there is no section Entitled "History" in the Document, create one stating the title, year, authors, and publisher of the Document as given on its Title Page, then add an item describing the Modified Version as stated in the previous sentence. J. Preserve the network location, if any, given in the Document for public access to a Transparent copy of the Document, and likewise the network locations given in the Document for previous versions it was based on. These may be placed in the "History" section. You may omit a network location for a work that was published at least four years before the Document itself, or if the original publisher of the version it refers to gives permission. K. For any section Entitled "Acknowledgements" or "Dedications", Preserve the Title of the section, and preserve in the section all the substance and tone of each of the contributor acknowledgements and/or dedications given therein. L. Preserve all the Invariant Sections of the Document, unaltered in their text and in their titles. Section numbers or the equivalent are not considered part of the section titles. M. Delete any section Entitled "Endorsements". Such a section may not be included in the Modified Version. N. Do not retitle any existing section to be Entitled "Endorsements" or to conflict in title with any Invariant Section. O. Preserve any Warranty Disclaimers. If the Modified Version includes new front-matter sections or appendices that qualify as Secondary Sections and contain no material copied from the Document, you may at your option designate some or all of these sections as invariant. To do this, add their titles to the list of Invariant Sections in the Modified Version's license notice. These titles must be distinct from any other section titles. You may add a section Entitled "Endorsements", provided it contains nothing but endorsements of your Modified Version by various parties--for example, statements of peer review or that the text has been approved by an organization as the authoritative definition of a standard. You may add a passage of up to five words as a Front-Cover Text, and a passage of up to 25 words as a Back-Cover Text, to the end of the list of Cover Texts in the Modified Version. Only one passage of Front-Cover Text and one of Back-Cover Text may be added by (or through arrangements made by) any one entity. If the Document already includes a cover text for the same cover, previously added by you or by arrangement made by the same entity you are acting on behalf of, you may not add another; but you may replace the old one, on explicit permission from the previous publisher that added the old one. The author(s) and publisher(s) of the Document do not by this License give permission to use their names for publicity for or to assert or imply endorsement of any Modified Version.

5. COMBINING DOCUMENTS

You may combine the Document with other documents released under this License, under the terms defined in section 4 above for modified versions, provided that you include in the combination all of the Invariant Sections of all of the original documents, unmodified, and list them all as Invariant Sections of your combined work in its license notice, and that you preserve all their Warranty Disclaimers. The combined work need only contain one copy of this License, and multiple identical Invariant Sections may be replaced with a single copy. If there are multiple Invariant Sections with the same name but different contents, make the title of each such section unique by adding at the end of it, in parentheses, the name of the original author or publisher of that section if known, or else a unique number. Make the same adjustment to the section titles in the list of Invariant Sections in the license notice of the combined work. In the combination, you must combine any sections Entitled "History" in the various original documents, forming one section Entitled "History"; likewise combine any sections Entitled "Acknowledgements", and any sections Entitled "Dedications". You must delete all sections Entitled "Endorsements".

6. COLLECTIONS OF DOCUMENTS

You may make a collection consisting of the Document and other documents released under this License, and replace the individual copies of this License in the various documents with a single copy that is included in the collection, provided that you follow the rules of this License for verbatim copying of each of the documents in all other respects. You may extract a single document from such a collection, and distribute it individually under this License, provided you insert a copy of this License into the extracted document, and follow this License in all other respects regarding verbatim copying of that document.

7. AGGREGATION WITH INDEPENDENT WORKS

A compilation of the Document or its derivatives with other separate and independent documents or works, in or on a volume of a storage or distribution medium, is called an "aggregate" if the copyright resulting from the compilation is not used to limit the legal rights of the compilation's users beyond what the individual works permit. When the Document is included in an aggregate, this License does not apply to the other works in the aggregate which are not themselves derivative works of the Document. If the Cover Text requirement of section 3 is applicable to these copies of the Document, then if the Document is less than one half of the entire aggregate, the Document's Cover Texts may be placed on covers that bracket the Document within the aggregate, or the electronic equivalent of covers if the Document is in electronic form. Otherwise they must appear on printed covers that bracket the whole aggregate.

8. TRANSLATION

Translation is considered a kind of modification, so you may distribute translations of the Document under the terms of section 4. Replacing Invariant Sections with translations requires special permission from their copyright holders, but you may include translations of some or all Invariant Sections in addition to the original versions of these Invariant Sections. You may include a translation of this License, and all the license notices in the Document, and any Warranty Disclaimers, provided that you also include the original English version of this License and the original versions of those notices and disclaimers. In case of a disagreement between the translation and the original version of this License or a notice or disclaimer, the original version will prevail. If a section in the Document is Entitled "Acknowledgements", "Dedications", or "History", the requirement (section 4) to Preserve its Title (section 1) will typically require changing the actual title.

9. TERMINATION

You may not copy, modify, sublicense, or distribute the Document except as expressly provided for under this License. Any other attempt to copy, modify, sublicense or distribute the Document is void, and will automatically terminate your rights under this License. However, parties who have received copies, or rights, from you under this License will not have their licenses terminated so long as such parties remain in full compliance.

10. FUTURE REVISIONS OF THIS LICENSE

The Free Software Foundation may publish new, revised versions of the GNU Free Documentation License from time to time. Such new versions will be similar in spirit to the present version, but may differ in detail to address new problems or concerns. See http://www.gnu.org/copyleft/. Each version of the License is given a distinguishing version number. If the Document specifies that a particular numbered version of this License "or any later version" applies to it, you have the option of following the terms and conditions either of that specified version or of any later version that has been published (not as a draft) by the Free Software Foundation. If the Document does not specify a version number of this License, you may choose any version ever published (not as a draft) by the Free Software Foundation. ADDENDUM: How to use this License for your documents To use this License in a document you have written, include a copy of the License in the document and put the following copyright and license notices just after the title page: Copyright (c) YEAR YOUR NAME. Permission is granted to copy, distribute and/or modify this document under the terms of the GNU Free Documentation License, Version 1.2 or any later version published by the Free Software Foundation; with no Invariant Sections, no Front-Cover Texts, and no Back-Cover Texts. A copy of the license is included in the section entitled "GNU Free Documentation License". If you have Invariant Sections, Front-Cover Texts and Back-Cover Texts, replace the "with...Texts." line with this: with the Invariant Sections being LIST THEIR TITLES, with the Front-Cover Texts being LIST, and with the Back-Cover Texts being LIST. If you have Invariant Sections without Cover Texts, or some other combination of the three, merge those two alternatives to suit the situation. If your document contains nontrivial examples of program code, we recommend releasing these examples in parallel under your choice of free software license, such as the GNU General Public License, to permit their use in free software.

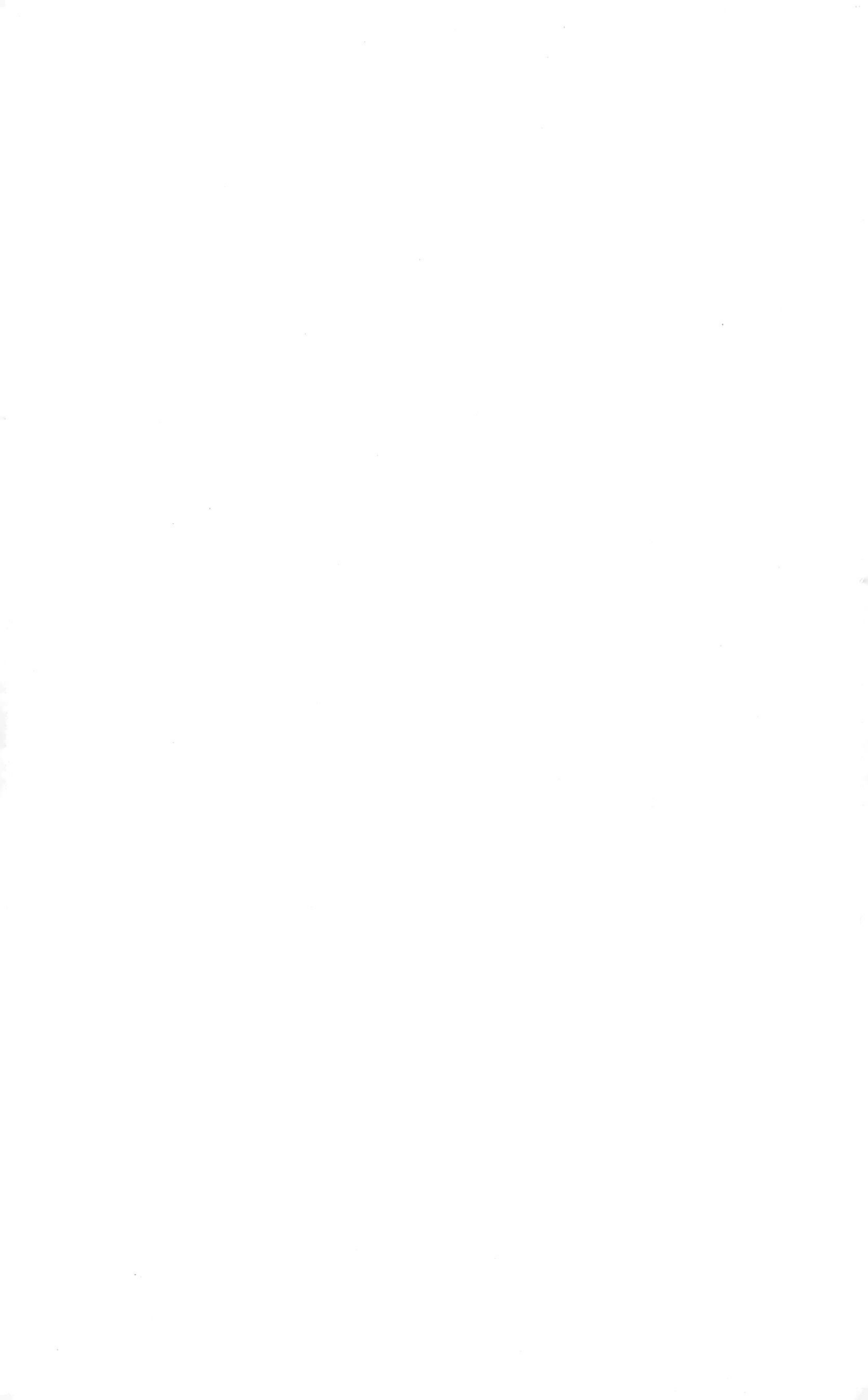